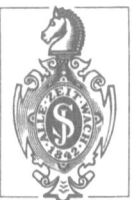

Clinical Practice in Urology
Series Editor: Geoffrey D. Chisholm

Chemotherapy and Urological Malignancy

Edited by
A.S.D. Spiers

Springer-Verlag
Berlin Heidelberg New York 1982

A. S. D. Spiers, MB, BS, MD(Melb.), PhD, FRCPE, FRACP, FACP
Professor of Medicine,
Division of Oncology,
The Albany Medical College,
Albany, New York 12208, USA.

Series Editor
Geoffrey D. Chisholm, ChM, FRCS, FRCSEd
Professor of Surgery,
University of Edinburgh,
Scotland.

Library of Congress Cataloging in Publication Data
Main entry under title: Chemotherapy and urological malignancy. (Clinical practice in urology). Bibliography: p. Includes index. 1. Genito-urinary organs – Chemotherapy. 2. Antineoplastic agents. I. Spiers, A.S.D. (Alexander Stewart Donaldson), 1936– . II. Series. [DNLM: 1. Genital neoplasms, Male – Drug therapy. 2. Urological neoplasms – Drug therapy. WJ 160 C517] RC280.G4C48 616.99′46061 82-5666
    ISBN-13: 978-1-4471-1334-8   e-ISBN-13: 978-1-4471-1332-4
    DOI: 10.1007/ 978-1-4471-1332-4

2128/3916-543210

To Albert Gordon Baikie, 1925–1975.
MB, ChB, DPA(Glas), FRCPEd, FRACP,
FRCPA, Foundation Professor of Medicine in
the University of Tasmania, Australia.

A friend and teacher to whom I am forever
indebted.

A.S.D.S. 1982

Series Editor's Foreword

Chemotherapy for malignant disease has brought about many rapid and often spectacular improvements in the survival rate of some groups of patients. Yet enthusiasm for these successes has, in part, been offset by the problems in evaluating responses to treatment and by the disappointment of failing to check the progress of still so many other tumours. These reactions will be no surprise to the medical historian but perhaps the expectations from scientific progress nowadays sometimes demand more than can reasonably be expected.

Another expectation is that any review of chemotherapy is completely up to date, even prophetic. Such is the expansion of the subject that new drugs and trial results are continually being reported but it is this very mass of information that creates its own problems and makes many clinicians despair of finding a balanced judgement on all of this information.

This was the challenge accepted by Professor Spiers. He then gathered together a group of colleagues who are amongst the acknowledged leaders in the field of chemotherapy for urological tumours, all of whom have made important contributions to this subject. However, each chapter is not merely a record of the author's experience but encompasses an assessment of past and present practice as well as perspectives in diagnosis and management. Almost all chapters include reference to published work up to and including 1981.

This book systematically reviews the role of chemotherapy for each of the anatomical sites that comprise the genito-urinary tract, including the adrenal gland. The successes and failures, rewards and frustrations that are part of the progress of chemotherapy are all encompassed by this group of tumours. Even where the progress has been dismal, it is important to appreciate the efforts that have been made and the problems that have beset many a study. The contributors have not avoided these issues and their presentation of all their experiences adds only to the appreciation of their successes.

Clinical trials have become the basis for all chemotherapeutic studies. Uncontrolled use of these powerful and often dangerous drugs is to be deplored. Collaborative studies both in the US and Europe are described in the hope that many readers will be encouraged not only to see that their patients receive the optimum treatment but also to participate in trials where the issues are far from resolved. Even where a treatment protocol has been well established, it will be evident that much of the success lies in careful patient monitoring. In this book, the contributors have carefully presented each subject so that the reader can judge what is the role of chemotherapy as part of overall management, what has become accepted clinical practice and what needs further evaluation.

Professor Spiers has met easily the challenge presented to him: this book offers the clinician a clear, concise and current summation of the state of the art and science of chemotherapy for urological tumours. The reader will readily appreciate the expertise with which the book has been prepared and will welcome the guidance offered herein.

Edinburgh, April 1982   Geoffrey Chisholm

Preface

The practising urologist spends much time as a specialized surgical oncologist. Although a minority of his patients have cancers, their needs for primary treatment, follow-up, reoperation, reconstructive and diversionary procedures, and continuing care, require from him a major commitment. In some other cancers, ongoing care can be assumed by the medical oncologist or the radiotherapist, but in urological malignancies, continuing surgical interventions are frequently necessary for the proper management of patients.

The most common urological cancers, those of the prostate and of the urothelium, are usually diagnosed by the urologist, who is then responsible for staging procedures and for the initial surgical management. There is an increasing tendency to involve the radiotherapist and the medical oncologist at an early stage in treatment planning, even in cases where primary surgical cure is likely. This admirable tendency has sprung from the willingness of urologists to support a multidisciplinary team approach to cancer. Its benefits include not only better care for patients, but also a widening of the experience of his colleagues in the other disciplines, who in the past were apt to see urological cancers only in their advanced stages.

The late complications of urological cancers, and the sequelae of treatment, often require the urologist's skills. His role as a surgical oncologist does not of course end there. As a medical oncologist, I find that the urology team is one of my most frequent allies, and many of my patients with tumors of nonurologic origin causing ureteric obstruction, have had extra months or years of useful life as a result of successful urinary diversion.

The aim of this book is to review the present status of chemotherapy for the common, and also the rare, urological cancers. For the urologist who may not himself administer chemotherapy, the aim is to provide an indication of what his medical oncologist colleague can offer. For the medical oncologist, we have endeavoured to provide both practical advice on current therapy and an indication of possible future progress. Of necessity, the authors have not confined themselves to a discussion of chemotherapy alone. Each chapter makes reference to diagnosis, pathology, staging, and natural history, and usually to surgical treatment and radiotherapy. This is a hallmark of progress:

chemotherapy for cancers cannot be considered in vacuo, but must be seen in the context of the extent and bulk of tumor, and of the contributions that can be made by other treatments. This multimodality approach to the treatment of cancer is emphasized throughout the book: in Wilms' tumor and in testicular cancer it has been dramatically successful, and it can reasonably be hoped to improve the outcome in commoner and more obdurate tumors such as bladder and prostatic cancer.

The subject matter is arranged on an obvious anatomical scheme beginning with the adrenal and proceeding downward to the testes. Drs. Zeffren and Yagoda have assembled the most comprehensive account extant of the drug therapy of adrenal cancer. Mitotane, the drug most widely used for this tumor, is unique among the cytoxic agents both for its peculiar specificity and its dual mechanism of action, antagonizing hormone synthesis and also inducing tumor cell necrosis. The development of better assays for both the drug and for the hormonal products of adrenal tumors promises to improve the management of this disease. The authors point out — and the theme recurs in other chapters — that the difficulties in the assessment of tumor response and the lack of adequately standardized criteria for reporting responses continue to impede progress in chemotherapy.

The two following chapters contrast sharply. Carcinoma of the kidney is remarkably resistant to cytotoxic drugs, and response to hormonal manipulations is uncommon, incomplete, usually of brief duration, and has not convincingly been shown to improve the length or quality of life. It is notable that recent studies, with proper evaluation of results, show the lowest response rates. There is a need for continuing cooperative studies to evaluate the many old and new drugs that have not undergone adequate trial in this neoplasm. In Wilms' tumor, Dr. Kumar and his colleagues tell a story of considerable achievement. In about forty years, the cure rate has risen from around 15% to about 90%. These impressive results are brought about by the successful application of multidisciplinary teamwork to the management of each patient. In Wilms' tumor, therapy has reached the encouraging stage where the overall intensity of the treatment actually is being reduced in some cases, because the risk of tumor recurrence is becoming less than the hazards of overtreatment.

Dr. Kasimis discusses the chemotherapy of the rarer tumors of the urothelium. His careful review underlines the paucity of data and the need for cooperative group studies to provide information that is unlikely to be gathered by a single institution. The results of surgery or radiotherapy are unsatisfactory, particularly for advanced tumors of the upper urothelial tract, and it cannot safely be assumed that agents with some activity against bladder cancer will be effective in pelvic, ureteric, or urethral tumors.

Superficial tumors of the urinary bladder possess many special features. Their tendency to recurrence and to multiplicity presents special problems to the surgeon who wishes to avoid cystectomy but does not wish to jeopardize the patients' survival. The accessibility of the bladder to repeated inspection and to endoscopic manipulations makes possible follow-up observation and treatment which is not feasible for the majority of visceral tumors. Topical therapy of early tumors, by the intravesical instillation of a variety of cytotoxic agents, is a logical and important approach to superficial bladder cancers. Dr. Soloway provides an outstanding review of the current status of intravesical therapy, and makes clear the many problems in this field which can be resolved only by carefully planned prospective clinical studies. Not least of the problems is the considerable expense of repeated cytoscopic examinations and the high cost of several of the cytotoxic agents employed. Such factors make it even more important that the value of intravesical therapy be critically assessed before it is too widely adopted.

Although advanced cancer of the bladder is more responsive to systemic chemotherapy than is renal cancer, existing chemotherapy regimens are rarely curative. Dr. Yagoda considers several agents, notably cisplatin, to be clinically useful, and there is evidence of prolongation of life for approximately a year in patients who respond to therapy. The role of adjuvant chemotherapy after apparently complete surgical resection of bladder cancers is being studied in randomized controlled trials. The need for effective adjuvant chemotherapy is undoubted, as over 50% of patients who are treated with radiotherapy followed by radical cystectomy die within 5 years from recurrent cancer.

Drs. Torti and Carter review the therapy of cancer of the prostate. A complex staging system now in use may enable better identification of poor prognostic groups. Although cancer of the prostate is common, there is surprisingly little reliable information on the effectiveness of cytotoxic drugs. In part this may be due to unwillingness to administer aggressive therapy to elderly men who frequently suffer from multiple medical illnesses. Undoubtedly, the widespread use of estrogens has for many years retarded research with other forms of drug therapy. Patients who receive cytotoxic drugs only after a prolonged trial of estrogens generally are in poor condition, with a high tumor burden, and are unlikely to achieve useful remissions with available agents. At least six drugs appear to have significant activity in prostatic cancer, but there is insufficient evidence to support their use in combinations, other than in the setting of a formal clinical study. The limitations of orchiectomy and the morbidity associated with the use of estrogens should prompt further trials of chemotherapy early in the course of metastatic cancer of the prostate.

Penile cancer is of interest to the chemotherapist because of its sometimes dramatic responsiveness to bleomycin, a sensitivity which unfortunately is not shared by other squamous cell cancers. Drs. Sklaroff and Yagoda consider bleomycin, methotrexate, and cisplatin to have useful activity in penile cancer; combined drug regimens are not yet adequately evaluated, and the value of adjuvant chemotherapy after surgery remains to be established. Very few institutions have sufficient patients to mount their own trials in this uncommon tumor, and cooperative multicenter studies are needed.

Drs. Einhorn and Williams review the management of testicular cancer. In the past decade there have been truly exciting advances in this field. The cure rate for disseminated testicular cancer has risen from approximately 10% to 70% with a combination of multiple-drug chemotherapy and, in some cases, surgical excision of residual disease.

Testicular cancer is a model of how progress can be made in cancer therapy. There have been improvements in the pathological characterization of the tumors, and lymphography and abdominal computerized axial tomography have greatly improved the staging of disease and the planning of therapy. Exploitation of the tumor markers, alpha fetoprotein and beta-chain human chorionic gonadotrophin, has enabled the monitoring of responses to therapy and the detection of residual disease with a refinement available in very few other tumors. The application of accurate staging, serial marker studies, and combinations of surgery and multiple-agent chemotherapy, has drastically improved the prognosis of this important tumor of young men.

Modern clinical studies in cancer frequently ask difficult questions and seek statistically secure answers. When relatively small differences in outcome are sought, large numbers of patients must be studied, and cooperative ventures involving many hospitals are essential if answers are to be provided in reasonably short periods of time. In the United States, cooperative groups have a long and distinguished history, but most do not extend across national boundaries. In Europe, the EORTC is an outstanding example of international cooperation in clinical cancer research. The work of the EORTC in urological cancers has been accorded a special chapter, because its emphasis, and in some instances its philosophy, often differ significantly from practice in the United States. Thus in testicular cancer, the approach to retroperitoneal nodes seems quite different on the two sides of the Atlantic, and it is uncertain if the 'correct' course of action has yet been defined. Perchance it is waiting to be picked up in mid-ocean.

It should give considerable satisfaction to the practising urologist that two urological cancers — Wilms' tumor and testicular cancer — are now repeatedly cited as examples of the success of modern cancer therapy, and as vindications of the multimodality approach to the management of tumors. Tomorrow's challenge is to lengthen the list.

Albany, April 1982   A. S. D. Spiers
                                            MD, PhD, FRCPEd, FRACP, FACP

Contents

Contributors

J. E. Champion, MD
Research Associate in Pediatric Hematology/Oncology,
St Jude Children's Research Hospital,
P.O. Box 318, Memphis,
Tennessee 38101, USA

S. K. Carter, MD
Director, Northern California Cancer Program,
P.O. Box 10144, Palo Alto,
California 94303, USA.
Clinical Professor of Medicine, University of California,
San Francisco
Consulting Professor of Medicine, Stanford University

M. de Pauw
Data Manager, EORTC Data Centre,
Institut Jules Bordet,
Brussels, Belgium

L. H. Einhorn, MD
Professor of Medicine,
Indiana University School of Medicine,
1100 West Michigan Street, Indianapolis,
Indiana 46223, USA

B. S. Kasimis, MD
Assistant Professor of Medicine,
Hematology/Oncology Section,
Veterans Administration Medical Centre,
5901 East Seventh Street, Long Beach,
California 90801, USA

A. P. M. Kumar, MD
Chief, Division of Surgery,
St Jude Children's Research Hospital,
P.O. Box 318, Memphis,
Tennessee 38101, USA

M. Pavone-Macaluso, MD
Professor and Chairman, Department of Urology,
University of Palermo, School of Medicine,
Palermo, Italy
Chairman, EORTC Urological Group

R. Sklaroff, MD
Fellow, Department of Hematology-Oncology,
Hahnemann Medical College and Hospital,
230 North Broad Street, Philadelphia,
Pennsylvania 19102, USA

P. H. Smith, MB, FRCS
Consultant Urological Surgeon,
St. James' University Hospital,
Leeds, Yorks., England

M. S. Soloway, MD
Professor, Department of Urology,
University of Tennessee Center for the Health Sciences,
Memphis, Tennessee, USA

A. S. D. Spiers, MD, PhD, FRCPEd, FRACP, FACP
Professor of Medicine, Division of Oncology,
The Albany Medical College, Albany,
New York 12208, USA

G. Stoter,
Medical Oncologist, Department of Oncology,
The Free University Hospital,
Amsterdam, The Netherlands
Chairman, Chemotherapy Committee, EORTC Urological
Group

R. Sylvester,
Assistant Director, EORTC Data Centre,
Institut Jules Bordet,
Brussels, Belgium

F. M. Torti, MD
Executive Officer, Northern California Oncology Group,
P.O. Box 10144, Palo Alto,
California 94303, USA
Associate Director for Clinical Activities, Northern California
Cancer Program
Assistant Professor of Medicine, Stanford University

J. Wilimas, MD
Assistant Member in Pediatric Hematology/Oncology,
St Jude Children's Research Hospital,
P.O. Box 318, Memphis,
Tennessee 38101, USA

S. D. Williams, MD
Assistant Professor of Medicine,
Indiana University School of Medicine,
1100 West Michigan Street, Indianapolis,
Indiana 46223, USA

A. Yagoda, MD
Associate Attending Physician,
Memorial Sloan–Kettering Cancer Center,
1275 York Avenue, New York,
New York 10021, USA

J. Zeffren, MD
Fellow, Solid Tumor Service,
Memorial Sloan–Kettering Cancer Center,
1275 York Avenue, New York,
New York 10021, USA

Chapter 1

Chemotherapy of Adrenal Cortical Carcinoma

J. Zeffren and A. Yagoda

The evaluation of anti-neoplastic agents in the treatment of patients with carcinoma of the adrenal cortex has been relatively limited since the incidence of this tumor is only 0.2/100,000. However, the propensity for adrenal cortical carcinoma to excrete hormones has led to unique groups of drugs which produce significant palliation of bothersome and life-threatening endocrinologically induced symptoms. Cushing's syndrome, virilization, feminization, sexual precocity, gynecomastia, hirsutism and hypertension, which are more frequently recognized in females and young children, are secondary to the overproduction of various class II (glucocorticoid) and III (17-ketosteroid) steroids. Malignant adrenal cell carcinoma, which is of mesodermal origin, does not excrete 'unusual steroids', rather they simply 'reflect inefficient use of the normal steroid precursors by the neoplasm and increased excretion of the metabolites normally present in only trace amounts' (Lipsett et al. 1963). For example, it has been estimated that the excretion rate of 17-hydroxycorticoids (17-OH) averages 1 mg/g of normal adrenal tissue compared to only 0.1–0.2 mg/g of tumor (Lipsett et al. 1963). In addition, such tumors are not totally independent of normal hormonal control since some investigators have found modulation of steroid secretion with ACTH (adrenocorticotropin) and dexamethasone administration (Rayfield et al. 1971; Bulger and Correa 1977). Thus, a large tumor burden is generally required before significant endocrinologic signs and symptoms appear which is in marked contrast to the efficient steroid production by small non-malignant adrenal cortical adenomas.

Typically, it is secondary effects of excessive steroid production that bring the patient to medical attention, which explains why in almost half the cases a palpable mass is discovered on initial physical examination (Lipsett et al. 1963; Hutter and Kayhoe 1966a). In a report from Memorial Sloan-Kettering Cancer Center, tumor size varied from 4 to 40 cm in diameter and only 1 of 34 cases showed gross evidence of encapsulation (Huvos et al. 1970). In another study (Lipsett et al. 1963) 20 of 38 patients had a tumor weighing >500 g. Local tumor extension is frequent as shown in a series of 127 cases in which 65% had tumor involvement of adjacent structures (Hutter and Kayhoe 1966a). Metastases are more frequently found in lung, liver, lymph nodes and intra-abdominally, and less commonly in skin, brain and osseous

Supported in part by Public Health Service grant CA-05826 and contract NO1-CM-57043 (Division of Cancer Treatment) from the National Cancer Institute, National Institutes of Health, Department of Health, Education and Welfare.

sites. Large masses, particularly abdominal metastases, tend to have areas of central necrosis.

Adrenal cortical carcinomas are divided into two groups — functioning and non-functioning — on a clinical and/or a biochemical basis. However, with modern biochemical techniques more tumors have been found to secrete into the blood various steroid metabolites not previously detected in the analysis of steroids excreted in urine. Such recent findings hinder an accurate assessment of the efficacy of some drugs in earlier trials.

Surgical resection is the treatment of choice for localized tumors. Even in selected patients with metastases, particularly those with Cushing's syndrome, significant palliation and possible prolongation of life can be achieved with surgery. However, palliation is short-lived in the majority of cases which present with metastases. In spite of a report by Steward et al. (1974) who noted beneficial effects with radiation therapy, most studies find these tumors relatively radioresistant. In addition, there is no evidence that post-operative irradiation decreases the incidence of metastases (Lipsett et al. 1963).

In late 1948 toxicologic studies in dogs described necrosis of the liver and adrenal cortex with the insecticide DDD, a chemical congener of DDT. The ortho, para isomer, o,p'-DDD (1, 1 dichloro 2 (o-chlorophenyl)-2-(p-chlorophenyl) ethane) was discovered to cause focal degeneration of the zona fasciculata and zona reticularis in the canine adrenal and eventually, o,p'-DDD was brought into clinical trials specifically for the treatment of metastatic tumors of the adrenal cortex.

In humans, 11-beta hydroxylation of adrenal steroids is blocked by daily doses of 0.5–3.0 g of o,p'-DDD and adrenal atrophy with glucocorticoid, and mineralocorticoid deficiency occurs with doses exceeding 3.0 g (Hogan et al. 1978). After an oral dose of o,p'-DDD approximately 40% is absorbed. Maximum plasma concentration is attained by 3–5 h and tissue (particularly in fat) equilibrium by 12 h. While 10% is excreted in urine as various metabolites, 20%–30% is stored in tissues as dichloroethene and acetic acid metabolites for 3.5–8.5+ months. Storage of o,p'DDD metabolites in fat is probably very prolonged since trace levels in plasma have been found 18 months after cessation of therapy (Hogan et al. 1978).

o,p'-DDD affects hepatic microsomes as shown by a change in the metabolism of barbiturates. Of clinical importance is the observation by Wortsman and Soler (1977) of an antagonism between spironolactones (e.g. Aldactone) and o,p'-DDD. In dogs, pretreatment with a spironolactone prevents o,p'-DDD-induced adrenocortical tissue necrosis. In humans, o,p'-DDD is ineffective, when given with spironolactone, in decreasing serum steroid levels and in ameliorating the symptoms of Cushing's syndrome.

The efficacy of o,p'-DDD has been established in a series of reports (Lipsett et al. 1963; Hutter and Kayhoe 1966a, 1966b; Lubitz et al. 1973) between 1959 and 1973 by the National Cancer Institute from data filed by over 200 physicians who administered the drug to patients with adrenal cortical carcinoma. In 1960, Bergenstal et al. described objective tumor regression and a decrease in abnormally elevated urinary steroid excretion in 7 of 18 patients given 8–10 g p.o. for 4–8 weeks. In the report by Hutter and Kayhoe (1966b) on 138 patients o,p'-DDD produced clinical responses in 35%. Tumor regression was obtained in 34% of 59 evaluable cases, but as noted by the authors 'exact measurements were rarely reported, a clear indication by the investigator of definite regression in measurable disease was accepted as evidence of response'. Reduction in elevated urinary 17-ketosteroids and 17-hydroxy or ketogenic steroids was found in 72% of 62 cases with response graded as good (30%–50% reduction of the metabolite measured) in 3% and 5%, respectively. In females, prolongation of life was found in o,p'-DDD responders who had documented tumor regression. Non-responders and patients who showed only a decrease in steroid excretion had a similar duration of survival. Age, site of metastases or the induction of toxic side effects with o,p'-DDD did not influence response. In patients with measurable lesions, although the response rate was 20% (2/10) for non-functioning tumors vs. 35% (12/34) for functioning tumors, the difference was not statistically significant ($p > 0.5$). In 115 patients treated between 1965 and 1969 Lubitz et al. (1973) noted tumor regression in 61% of 75 cases and a decrease in elevated steroid excretion in 85% of 61 cases. Increased survival occurred primarily in responders who had measurable tumor. Some patients who relapsed after chemotherapy was discontinued because of toxicity experienced a second objective remission with resumption of o,p'-DDD. The reason for the higher response rate in the summary of trials reported by Lubitz et al. (1973) compared with Hutter and Kayhoe (1966b) could be explained by patient selection (i.e. a shorter interval between diagnosis and treatment), different histologic types (Huvos et al. 1970) varied drug dosages and durations of therapy, assessment of changes in tumor volume (by 95 different physicians) and more accurate biochemical tests coupled with a response criterion of *only* a greater than 30% reduction in urinary steroid excretion, equal to the 'fair' category in the series of Hutter and Kayhoe (1966b).

The longest duration of survival has been reported by Becker and Schumacher (1975) and Exelby (1975) who describe two patients alive at 4 and 7 years, and one patient alive at 6 years, respectively, after beginning o,p'-DDD therapy. However, there are two negative reports by Hajjer et al. (1975) and Bulger and Correa (1977). In the former study, a small group of patients obtained no benefit with the use of o,p'-DDD as an adjunct to surgery or as a single therapy, while in the latter, no responses were observed in five patients, but 'in all but one patient the drug was discontinued in less than 1 month because of poor patient tolerance'.

Between 1949 and 1977 twelve patients at Memorial Sloan-Kettering Cancer Center were given o,p'-DDD alone. Doses, schedules and the duration of drug administration varied. Of nine adequately treated patients one obtained complete remission and one a minor response. An additional patient who received o,p'-DDD combined with a 4-month course of 5-fluorouracil has remained in complete remission for 3+ years.

The onset of biochemical response to daily administration of o,p'-DDD is rapid; 50% by day 17 in one series (Lubitz et al. 1973), and 49% within 21 days and 37% between 21–30 days in another series (Hutter and Kayhoe 1966b). Measurable tumor regression occurs later, 4–6 weeks (range 1½–28 weeks) with a mean of 8–9 weeks. Occasionally, responses can be very delayed with initial improvement observed biochemically at 2.5 months and on physical examination at 19 months (Lubitz et al. 1973). Thus, the definition of an adequate trial of o,p'-DDD should be 4–6 weeks for biochemical parameters and 12 weeks for measurable lesions (Exelby 1975).

The proper dose, schedule and duration of therapy of o,p'-DDD is still undetermined. Since the major dose-limiting toxicities of o,p'-DDD are gastrointestinal disturbances — anorexia, nausea, vomiting and diarrhea and central nervous system abnormalities – depression ('gloom and doom'), lethargy, somnolence, vertigo and confusion, many patients refuse maintenance therapy. Hutter and Kayhoe (1966b) noted responses biochemically in 29 of 31 patients to doses of ≤ 10 g daily (average 8.5 g) and tumor regression in 15 patients with an average dose of 8.1 g daily. One patient who relapsed after a 20-month remission responded again when o,p'-DDD was increased from 4 to 8 g daily. Although response may have been dose-dependent in one or two patients, Hutter and Kayhoe (1966b) concluded that 'undesirable side effects of o,p'-DDD are not required for response'. Lubitz et al. (1973) cautioned against interrupting o,p'-DDD therapy.

Some patients exhibited rapid tumor exacerbation evidenced by an increase in urinary steroid levels and less effectiveness with subsequent retreatment. Bergenstal et al. (1960) recommended 10 g or more daily with re-adjustment to a maximally tolerated dose 3–7 days later. However, Hogan et al. (1978) who utilized plasma o,p'-DDD levels, estimated that initially 2 g daily followed by a slow dose escalation to 6 g daily was desirable. At Memorial Hospital, patients started on high doses frequently refused further therapy because of intense gastrointestinal symptoms. We recommend a starting dose of 2 g daily (four 500 mg tablets) followed by a slow dose escalation. Since steroid production is rapidly blocked by o,p'-DDD, all patients receive replacement steroids and many require mineralocorticoid replacement as well. In the future, the use of modern, sophisticated steroid and o,p'-DDD assays should assist physicians in titrating proper doses.

Does o,p'-DDD increase survival? The natural history of adrenal cortical carcinoma was described by MacFarlane (1958) who found only 24% (13/55) of patients alive 3 years after surgery; excluding postoperative deaths, the figure increased to 30%. In untreated patients the mean and median survival times from diagnosis to death were 2.9 and 2.5 months, respectively. Huvos et al. (1970) described mean survival times from diagnosis to death of 1.7 years for men and 2.6 years for women, while Hutter and Kayhoe (1966b) reported 38% of men and 52% of women alive at 4 years. In the series of Lubitz et al. (1973) non-responders (equal to the advanced disease presentation of the untreated group in MacFarlane's study) lived an average of 3 months vs. 10.3 months for responders, which is identical to the duration of response (10.2 months) reported by Hutter and Kayhoe (1966b). In addition, in female patients with measurable disease over 75% of responders vs. <50% of non-responders were alive at 44 months.

All trials indicate a favorable effect of o,p'-DDD on survival, particularly in females with measurable disease and tumor regression and in patients with non-functioning adrenal cortical carcinomas, i.e. undifferentiated, sarcomatous, and clear cell (resembling normal cells of the zona glomerulosa) tumors. Different response rates to o,p'-DDD can be attributed to histologic subtypes of adrenal cortical carcinoma.

Should o,p'-DDD be used in an adjuvant fashion? Lipsett et al. (1963) recommended intensive therapy with o,p'-DDD with increases in urinary 17-ketosteroid excretion but suggested that 'o,p'-DDD may be most successful in patients with the least disease'. Hutter and Kayhoe (1966b) suggested that o,p'-DDD be used only in 'patients for whom surgery is no longer indicated'. o,p'-DDD as adjuvant therapy was investigated in four patients all of whom survived 2–13+ years (Brown and Schumacher 1979). Of note, two patients who stopped therapy and eventually had tumor recurrence survived 3–3½ years. In nine children given o,p'-DDD prophylactically, four were alive 1+–8+ years later (Exelby 1975). At Memorial Sloan-Kettering Cancer Center all children are treated prophylactically after surgery. Lubitz et al. (1973) concluded that early treatment might enhance clinical response, and that 'while there is no data, it appears that prophylactic use of mitotane should be considered following surgery when there is uncertainty as to whether metastatic seeding has occurred'. Dose escalation of o,p'-DDD in an adjuvant setting is difficult, since most patients cannot tolerate more than 6 g daily for periods greater than 2 months. However, Hutter and Kayhoe (1966b) described 18 patients who tolerated therapy with dose modification for >1 year and three for >2 years. In a remarkable case a 7-year-old female was given o,p'-DDD maintenance, 7 g daily, for 5 years to a cumulative dose of 11 kg (Exelby 1975). Thus far, no long term side effects have been noted 2 years after cessation of therapy.

The occurrence of adrenal insufficiency in a child receiving an anti-convulsant,

Table 1.1. Single agent chemotherapeutic drug trials in adrenal cortical carcinoma

Drugs	References	No. of trials	CR	PR	MR	NR
Nitrogen mustard	MH	2				2
NCS 1026	MH	1				1
Ethionine	MH	1				1
Streptozotocin	Schein et al. 1974	1				1
Aminoglutethimide	Camacho et al. 1966; Kumar et al. 1969; Schteingart et al. 1966; Smilo et al. 1967	3				3
Dihydroxybusulfan	Dietrich 1968	1				1
5 Fluorouracil	Bulger and Correa 1977; Hajjar et al. 1975; Moore et al. 1968	3				3
Cyclocytidine	Burgess et al. 1977	1				1
Anguidine	Murphy et al. 1978	1				1
BCNU	Marsh et al. 1971; MH	2				2
Hexamethylmelamine	Bergevin et al. 1973	1				1
Hydrazine sulfate	Lerner and Regelson 1976	1				1
Adriamycin	Bulger and Correa 1977; Hajjar et al. 1975; O'Bryan et al. 1973	3				3
Triethylene thiophosphoramide	Bulger and Correa 1977; Hajjar et al. 1975	1				1
Megestrol	Bulger and Correa 1977; Hajjar et al. 1975	1				1
Cis-DDP	MH	2		1		1
P-208 + 6-MP	MH	1				1
Chlorambucil + vinblastine	MH	1				1
o,p'-DDD + 5-FU	Ostuni and Roginsky 1975	1	1			
BCNU + vincristine	Stolinsky et al. 1974	1				1
Adriamycin + bleomycin	Tormey et al. 1973	1		1		
Adriamycin + 5-FU	Bulger and Correa 1977; Hajjar et al. 1975	1				1
CCNU + vinblastine	Bulger and Correa 1977; Hajjar et al. 1975	1				1
Cyclophosphamide, vincristine, MeCCNU, bleomycin	Livingston et al. 1975	3			2	1
Cyclophosphamide, 5-FU, methotrexate, vincristine	Gerner and Moore 1973	3				3
Mitomycin-C + 5-FU	MH	1				1
Adriamycin + streptozotocin	MH	1				1
Cis-DDP + 5-FU	MH	1				1
Dacarbazine (DTIC)	MH	1	Inadequate trial			
Vinblastine, cyclophosphamide actinomycin-D, o,p'-DDD	MH	1	Inadequate trial			
Totals		43	1	2	2	36

MH = Memorial Hospital.
CR = Complete remission.
PR = Partial remission.
MR = Minor response.
NR = No response.

aminoglutethimide, prompted clinical trials in patients with metastatic adrenal cortical carcinoma (Comacho et al. 1966). Aminoglutethimide blocks all pathways of steroid synthesis thereby rapidly suppressing cortisol production by inhibition of 21-hydroxylation. However, no anti-tumor effect has been noted. Some investigators (Schteingart et al. 1966; Smilo et al. 1967; Kumar et al. 1969) have suggested the use of o,p'-DDD and aminoglutethimide together in order to minimize the toxicity of high doses of o,p'-DDD and more effectively alleviate Cushing's syndrome. Another agent which can produce adrenal suppression and has been used in the treatment of adrenal carcinoma is amphenidone (Hertz et al. 1956).

In an extensive review of all disease-oriented as well as drug-oriented phase I and II trials no single agent was found to be of consistent benefit (Table 1.1). Some reports were excluded because remissions were described without sufficient data to evaluate response criteria, drug dosages, metastatic sites, or adequacy of trial. All cases were evaluated by the following criteria: complete remission — disappearance of all measurable disease, partial remission — tumor regression of >50% for more than 1 month, and minor remission — 'significant objective regression' (as stated by some investigators) or tumor regression of 25%–50% for >1 month. All other categories were listed as progression of disease. In 40 chemotherapy trials in 38 patients culled from the literature and from histologically proven adult cases at Memorial Sloan-Kettering Cancer Center between 1949 and 1977, the only significant responses were an 11-month remission with methyl-mitomycin C (porfiromycin) (Izbicki et al. 1972) and a 6-month remission with cis-diamminedichloride platinum (II) (Mérrin 1979).

There have been scattered reports of combination therapy with o,p'-DDD and 5-fluorouracil or adriamycin. Ostuni and Roginsky (1975) used o,p'-DDD (469 g) and 5-fluorouracil (22.4 g) in a 17-year-old female with pulmonary and hepatic metastases. Treatment was administered over 4 months and re-evaluation revealed complete remission. The patient died 9 years later and post mortem examination revealed no evidence of adrenal cortical carcinoma. In another case at Memorial Hospital a patient who started on o,p'-DDD and 5-fluorouracil has been in complete remission for 3 years and without therapy for 1½ years. However, it is difficult to ascribe an additive or synergistic effect to o,p'-DDD combination regimens since o,p'-DDD alone is an active drug in adrenal cortical carcinoma.

Presently, o,p'-DDD remains the drug of choice. Doses between 2 and 8 g daily should be administered for a minimum of 3 months and patients who respond should be given the maximally tolerated dose. If o,p'-DDD is stopped and tumor recurs the drug should be re-started. Whether low doses of o,p'-DDD or an intermittent regimen would be as efficacious is unknown but all biologic parameters using the most sophisticated tests available should be followed to document response and titrate doses.

In the future, measurements of o,p'-DDD metabolites in blood or tissues may be useful in adjusting dosage. Although the evaluation of anti-neoplastic chemotherapeutic agents is limited, porfiromycin, cis-diamminedichloride platinum (II) and 5-fluorouracil may be of some benefit in advanced cases and in an adjuvant setting when combined with o,p'-DDD.

References

Becker D, Schumacher OP (1975) o,p'DDD therapy in invasive adrenocortical carcinoma. Ann Intern Med 82: 677–679

Bergenstal DM, Hertz R, Lipsett MB, Moy RH (1960) Chemotherapy of adrenocortical cancer with o,p'DDD. Ann Intern Med 53: 672

Bergevin PR, Tormey DC, Blom J (1973) Clinical evaluation of hexamethylmelamine. Cancer Chemother Rep 57: 51–58

Brown D, Schumacher OP (1979) Adjuvant therapy, o,p'DDD in the treatment of metastatic adreno-cortical carcinoma. Clin Res 27: 626a

Bulger AR, Correa RJ (1977) Experience with adrenal cortical carcinoma. Urology 10: 12–18

Burgess MA, Bodey GP, Minow RA, Gottlieb JA (1977) Phase I–II evaluation of cyclocytidine. Cancer Treat Rep 61: 437–443

Camacho A, Brough AJ, Cash R, Wilroy RS (1966) Adrenal toxicity associated with the administration of an anticonvulsant drug. J Pediatr 68: 852

Dietrich FS (1968) Clinical trial with dihydroxybusulfan. Cancer Chemother Rep 52: 603–609

Exelby PR (1975) Adrenal cortical carcinoma in a child. Clin Bull 5: 26–31

Gerner RE, Moore GE (1973) Multiple-drug therapy for malignant solid tumors in adults. Cancer Chemother Rep 57: 237–239

Hajjar RA, Hickey RC, Samaan NA (1975) Adrenal cortical carcinoma — A study of 32 patients. Cancer 35: 549–554

Harrison JH, Mahoney EM, Bennett AH (1973) Tumors of the adrenal cortex. Cancer 32: 1227–1235

Hertz R, Pittman JA, Graff MM (1956) Amphenidone: Toxicity and effects on adrenal and thyroid function in man. J Clin Endocrinol 16: 705

Hogan TF, Citirin DL, Johnson BM, Nakamura S, Davis TE, Borden EC (1978) o,p'DDD therapy of adrenal cortical carcinoma. Cancer 42: 2177–2181

Hutter AM Jr, Kayhoe DE (1966a) Adrenal cortical carcinoma — Clinical features of 138 patients. Am J Med 41: 572–580

Hutter AM Jr, Kayhoe DE (1966b) Adrenal cortical carcinoma — Results of treatment with o,p'DDD in 138 patients. Am J Med 41: 581–592

Huvos HG, Hajdu SI, Brasfield RD, Foote FW Jr (1970) Adrenal cortical carcinoma — Clinicopathologic study of 34 cases. Cancer 25: 354–361

Izbicki R, Al-Saraf M, Reed ML, Vaughn CB, Vaitkevicius VK (1972) Further clinical trials with porfiromycin (NSC-56410) (large intermittent doses). Cancer Chemother Rep 56: 615–624

Kumar RS, Kamitsuna S, Cole VW (1969) Aminoglutethimide in functioning adrenal carcinoma. South Med J 62: 225–227

Lerner HJ, Regelson W (1976) Clinical trial of hydrazine sulfate in solid tumors. Cancer Treat Rep 60: 959–960

Lipsett MB, Hertz R, Ross GT (1963) Clinical and pathophysiologic aspects of adrenocortical carcinoma. Am J Med 35: 374–383

Livingston RB, Einhorn LH, Bodey GP, Burgess MA, Freireich EJ, Gottlieb JA (1975) COMB (cyclo-phosphamide, Oncovin, methyl CCNU, and bleomycin): A four-drug combination in solid tumors. Cancer 36: 327–332

Lubitz JA, Freeman L, Okun R (1973) Mitotane use in inoperable adrenal cortical carcinoma. JAMA 223: 1109–1112

MacFarlane DA (1958) Cancer of the adrenal cortex. Ann R Coll Surg Engl 23: 155

Marsh JC, DeConti RC, Hubbard SP (1971) Treatment of Hodgkin's disease and other cancers with 1,3 BCNU. Cancer Chemother Rep 55: 599–606

Merrin CE (1979) Treatment of genitourinary tumors with cis-dichlorodiammine platinum(II): Experience in 250 patients. Cancer Treatment Rep 63: 1579–1584

Moore GE, Bross IDJ, Ausman R, Nadler S, Jones R Jr, Slack N, Rimm AA (1968) Effects of 5-fluorouracil in 389 patients with cancer. Cancer Chemother Rep 52: 641–653

Murphy WK, Burgess MA, Valdivieso M, Livingston RB, Bodey GP, Freireich EJ (1978) Phase I clinical evaluation of anguidine. Cancer Treat Rep 62: 1497–1502

O'Bryan RM, Luce JK, Talley RW, Gottlieb JA, Baker LH, Bonadonna G (1973) Phase II evaluation of adriamycin in human neoplasia. Cancer 32: 1–8

Ostuni JA, Roginsky MS (1975) Metastatic adrenal cortical carcinoma — documented cure with com-bined chemotherapy. Arch Intern Med 135: 1257–1258

Rayfield EJ, Rose LI, Cain JP, Dluhy RG, Williams GH (1971) ACTH-responsive, dexamethasone-suppressible adrenocortical carcinoma. N Engl J Med 284: 591–592

Schein PS, O'Connell MJ, Blom J, Hubbard S, Magrath IT, Bergevin P, Wiernik PH, Ziegler JL, DeVita VT (1974) Clinical antitumor activity and toxicity of streptozotocin. Cancer 34: 993–1000

Schteingart DE, Cash R, Conn JW (1966) Aminoglutethimide and metastatic adrenal cancer. JAMA 198: 1007

Smilo RP, Earll JM, Forsham PH (1967) Suppression of tumorous adrenal hyperfunction by amino-glutethimide. Metabolism 16: 374

Stewart DR, Morris-Jones PH, Jolleys A (1974) Carcinoma of the adrenal gland in children. J Pediatr Surg 9: 59–67

Stolinsky DC, Pugh RP, Bohannon RA, Bogdon DL, Bateman JR (1974) Clinical trial of BCNU combined with vincristine in disseminated gastrointestinal cancer and other neoplasms. Cancer Chemother Rep 58: 947–950
Tormey DC, Bergevin PR, Blom J, Petty W (1973) Preliminary trials with a combination of adriamycin and bleomycin in adult malignancies. Cancer Chemother Rep 57: 413–418
Wortsman J, Soler NG (1977) Mitotane–spironolactone antagonism in Cushing's disease. JAMA 238: 2527

The authors wish to acknowledge the secretarial assistance of Mrs. Isa Irvin.

Chapter 2

Cytotoxic Drugs and Hormonal Manipulations in the Management of Carcinoma of the Kidney

A. S. D. Spiers

Introduction

The commonest renal tumor in adults is that arising from the cells of renal parenchyma. These cancers were described by Grawitz (1883), who named them hypernephromas upon the supposition that they might arise from nests of adrenal tissue in the kidney. The names 'hypernephroma' and 'Grawitz tumor' are obsolete, and renal carcinoma (or renal cell carcinoma) is the most appropriate term, since the tumors arise from the secretory cells of the renal tubular epithelium. Renal carcinoma is not a common disease; its incidence is about 7.5 cases per 100,000 population. In the United States there are about 7000 deaths from this tumor each year (American Cancer Society 1973): this represents 2.3% of male cancer deaths and 1.6% of cancer deaths in women.

Although only a minor contributor to cancer mortality, carcinoma of the kidney has excited much interest in diverse fields of medicine. To the surgeon it presents both diagnostic problems and a therapeutic challenge. Its diagnosis has stimulated much research in radiology, with the development of advanced techniques in tomography, angiography, and ultrasonography. The internist encounters this neoplasm as an occasional cause of polycythemia and also of pyrexia of obscure origin. The occurrence of solitary pulmonary metastases and the propensity of renal carcinoma to involve the skeleton make this a tumor of interest to the thoracic surgeon and the orthopedic surgeon. Compression of the spinal cord and neuro-surgical intervention are not rare events. Radiotherapists frequently are called upon to palliate the patient with metastatic renal carcinoma but can contribute little to definitive treatment. For the medical oncologist, this tumor is both a frustration and a challenge. Renal carcinoma is an outstanding example of a tumor which usually is totally resistant to cytotoxic drugs. In the minority of cases that show some regression of tumor after drug therapy, it is uncertain whether survival is prolonged. Thus in renal carcinoma, the achievements of cancer chemotherapy are very slight: conversely, the opportunity to effect a major improvement in management is great. Recent scientific developments have the potential to make this much-needed improvement attainable.

Need for Effective Chemotherapy in Renal Carcinoma

The natural history of this tumor and the poor results of surgical treatment dictate the need for therapy effective in disseminated disease.

Pathology and Natural History

The histological picture varies both from one tumor to another and in different areas of the same tumor. A broad subdivision into clear cell tumors and granular cell tumors is possible, but the groups shade into one another and some tumors contain cells of both types in different areas. Granular cell tumors may have a worse prognosis (Prout 1973), but this is questionable. Three interrelated features are of prognostic importance: the histological structure of the tumor, the presence of capsular invasion, and infiltration of the renal veins (Carter 1968). Renal cancers tend to spread locally and later develop distant metastases; a useful staging system is that of Robson et al. (1969):
  1) Tumor confined to renal parenchyma;
  2) Extension beyond the kidney but within Gerota's fascia;
  3) Renal vein, inferior vena cava, or regional lymph node involvement;
  4) Adjacent organs other than adrenal involved, or distant metastases.

Results of Surgery

Robson's group found 5-year survivals of 66%, 64%, 42% and 11% in stages 1, 2, 3 and 4 respectively. Although almost a third of patients have metastatic disease before surgery, this proportion does not increase between stages 1 and 2 — thus invasion of the perinephric fat is not of serious import unless accompanied by vascular or lymphatic invasion. However, at least one-third of patients have advanced disease (stages 3 and 4) at presentation, with a greater than 60% likelihood of metastatic disease. The crude survival for all stages in Robson's series was 52% at 5 years and 48% at 10 years. The stage of disease at presentation, rather than the extent of the surgery performed, is the principal determinant of survival. Since there is no indication that patients with renal carcinoma are presenting earlier, and there is no screening procedure which is practicable for this uncommon tumor, it follows that the survival of patients with renal cancer requires some form of systemic therapy which will control or eradicate metastatic disease. The situation resembles that in breast cancer, with the important difference that comparably effective chemotherapy is not yet available.

Choice of Therapy

Surgery

Surgical exploration is usually required to establish the histologic diagnosis and is essential in most cases for staging of the tumor. Resection, if technically possible, is then carried out. The presence of Stage 4 disease, with clearly demonstrable metastases, does not preclude surgery if serious problems — fever, pain, hematuria — can be relieved by nephrectomy. The regression of documented metastases after nephrectomy is very rare (Middleton 1967; Prout 1973) and is not in itself an indication for removal of the primary tumor. Resection of the kidney tumor and removal of an apparently solitary metastasis has led to a 34% 5-year survival in one series (Prout 1973) but most patients with one apparent metastasis at the time of presentation in fact have multiple metastases. The prognosis apparently is much better when a single metastatic lesion appears months or years after nephrectomy.

Recently, some evidence has been presented that nephrectomy may be of value when performed as an adjunct to chemotherapy (Ishmael et al. 1980). Response rates in patients with metastatic disease treated with a combination of adriamycin, vincristine, medroxyprogesterone and BCG vaccine were reported to be higher in patients who had undergone nephrectomy. Eight of ten patients who had only pulmonary metastases responded when this chemotherapy was administered after nephrectomy. These results require confirmation, as the study apparently was not randomized and the possibility exists that there was patient selection, nephrectomy not being performed in the patients with more extensive metastatic disease and worse general condition. Meanwhile, the place of adjunctive nephrectomy in the absence of symptoms from the primary tumor such as pain or haematuria remains uncertain.

Radiotherapy

Carcinoma of the kidney is relatively radioresistant. Radiotherapy is valuable in the palliative treatment of metastases — e.g. in bone or brain, or in the lung with resultant hemoptysis — but has not found a place in primary treatment. There is no good evidence that preoperative or postoperative irradiation of the renal area improves the surgical cure rate.

Chemotherapy

For the patient with widely disseminated renal carcinoma, the therapeutic options are chemotherapy with cytotoxic drugs and hormonal agents, or symptomatic treatment with analgesics and psychotropic drugs. As will be seen, the benefits of chemotherapy are uncommon in occurrence and small in extent, while toxicity often is considerable. Because it is relatively innocuous, hormonal therapy may be tried in most patients, the expectation of toxicity being even smaller than that of producing major benefit. In contrast, cytotoxic drug therapy usually is withheld unless there is symptomatic disease that cannot be relieved by surgery, radiotherapy, or hormones. In the absence of symptoms, chemotherapy occasionally is given because the patient requests that a trial of cytotoxic drugs be made. This is reasonable if the patient's nutritional state and bone marrow, hepatic, and renal function are adequate. Patients with massive disease, cachexia, and no compromise of renal, hepatic or hematopoietic function, and those with no measurable indices for the success or otherwise of therapy, should not receive aggressive drug therapy. A quite separate indication for chemotherapy is the patient with measurable metastatic disease who volunteers to participate in a formal study of an experimental agent — this is an investigative, rather than a therapeutic indication.

Strict adherence to the above criteria will avoid much morbidity and mortality, because intensive treatment will be withheld from those patients with advanced disease who cannot possibly benefit from it and who are most liable to the more serious complications of treatment.

Problems in Chemotherapy of Renal Carcinoma

Undoubtedly the greatest single obstacle to the chemotherapeutic control of renal cancer is the lack of any drugs with a high, or even an encouraging, success rate. Other factors which contribute to the problem are:

(a) the comparative rarity of the tumor, so that single institutions are unlikely to accrue significant series of patients in a reasonable time period;

(b) until recently, patients were apt to be managed surgically and by radiotherapy, and were unlikely to be seen by the medical oncologist until disease had become so advanced that a trial of chemotherapy frequently was precluded;

(c) the occurrence of 'spontaneous' regressions of disease, which bring temporary benefit to a minority of patients but also make it difficult to assess the efficacy of new drugs in this disease: there is always the suspicion that a small number of apparent 'therapeutic responses' may represent the occurrence of a few spontaneous regressions. This argument has indeed been advanced — perhaps correctly — when the results obtained with chemotherapy by one group cannot be reproduced by another group.

(d) the effect of chemotherapy upon survival is even more difficult to measure than its impact upon the size of measurable tumors. Patients with proved metastatic renal carcinoma may have a rapid downhill course and die in a few months; however, in some the course may be protracted, even for several years. Very late recurrence of renal cancer in patients who apparently were cured by surgery further confounds the evaluation of therapy (Kradjian and Bennington 1964).

The true incidence of spontaneous regression of renal cancer, like that of the regression of metastases from renal cancer after removal of the primary tumor, is uncertain. In both situations, the rare cases of regression are reported and the much commoner cases of progression and death are not. One can blame authors, editors and the natural optimism of human nature. It is certain that spontaneous regression does not intervene in the clinical course of most patients. Similarly, removal of the primary tumor is not justified when the only 'indication' is the optimistic idea that widely disseminated metastatic disease may then regress. That spontaneous regression does occur seems beyond doubt. Everson and Cole (1966) reviewed the world literature from 1900 and found 31 cases which they accepted as showing the spontaneous regression of renal cancer. The occurrence of such regression has, by some, been interpreted as possibly due to the operation of body defenses against tumors and has inspired attempts to eradicate renal cancer by some form of immunotherapy. These studies will be considered later.

Single-Agent Chemotherapy

A survey of the results of using individual cytotoxic drugs in patients with metastatic carcinoma of the kidney should give an accurate idea of the utility, or otherwise, of each agent and could suggest which drugs might be considered for study as components of a multi-agent regimen. Unfortunately, results as reported are not always readily compared. The criteria of tumor response vary from one group of investigators to another and also from one era to another; sometimes the criteria are not even specified. Very few reports enable the assessment of possible effects on patient *survival*, which is more important to the clinician, and the patient, than mere tumor shrinkage. Regression of tumor masses is not always accompanied by an increase in the quality or duration of the patient's life. There have been insufficient controlled studies which compare the survival of patients and the incidence of tumor shrinkage in a placebo group with the experience of patients who receive a potentially active drug. These limitations must be borne in mind in the following account.

Alkylating Agents

In 1967, Woodruff et al. reviewed the literature pertaining to chemotherapy in renal carcinoma. They reported a total of 53 cases treated with a variety of alkylating agents, with six objective responses (11%). Two of 15 patients treated with chlorambucil and 2 of 16 who received cyclophosphamide showed tumor regression. Talley (1973) treated 22 patients with a variety of alkylating agents and observed no responses. Lokich and Harrison (1975) found no tumor regressions in 14 patients treated with either mitomycin C, cyclophosphamide, or triethylene melamine. Even worse results were reported by Canadian workers, who saw no responses in ten patients treated with cyclophosphamide and considered that there was accelerated tumor growth in three patients (Kiruluta et al. 1975). Cyclophosphamide in high dose (40 mg/kg body weight every 3 weeks) recently was evaluated in ten patients (Wajsman et al. 1980). There were no objective responses and five patients showed progressive disease, and the authors rightly concluded that cyclophosphamide appeared valueless in metastatic renal carcinoma. The investigational alkylating agent dibromodulcitol was administered to 19 patients with four objective responses (Carter and Wasserman 1975).

No alkylating agent has undergone extensive trial in renal cancer, but the above partial survey of the literature discloses only ten responses in a total of 118 patients (8.5%). It is uncertain how much this figure exceeds the 'spontaneous' waxing and waning of metastatic lesions in this disease and it is impossible to determine whether life was prolonged or improved in quality for any of the ten responding patients. There is a need for more thorough trials of single alkylating agents (e.g. dibromo-dulcitol) but the dismal experience so far suggests that no clinically valuable agent may emerge from such studies.

Nitrosoureas

The nitrosoureas have been incompletely evaluated in carcinoma of the kidney, but experience to date is not encouraging. Mittelman et al. (1973) treated 23 patients with lomustine (CCNU): in 20 evaluable patients, objective remission lasting 3–6 months was seen in four and in a further two there was stabilization of disease for over 6 months. Apparent arrest of disease also occurs spontaneously in renal cancer and its occurence during chemotherapy consequently is unimpressive. Carter and Wasserman (1975) found responses in 4 of 59 patients treated with CCNU and none of 21 patients treated with methyl-CCNU. The overall response rate for these nitrosoureas thus was 4 of 80 (5%), and it seems very unlikely that a minimum 'acceptable' response rate (20%) could be achieved with more extensive trials. The newer nitrosoureas — e.g. streptozotocin — are insufficiently studied in renal cancer.

The Eastern Cooperative Oncology Group has completed a trial of piperidyl nitrosourea (PCNU) in renal carcinoma: this agent appears not to possess useful activity.

Antimetabolite Drugs

The pyrimidine antagonist 5-fluorouracil (5-FU) was reported to produce an objective response in 5 out of 36 patients (14%) by Woodruff et al. (1967). Talley (1973) found no responses in 12 patients, and this experience has been paralleled by our own. Carter and Wasserman's estimate (1975) of an 8% regression rate with 5-FU is similarly unimpressive.

Experience with other antimetabolite drugs is both fragmentary and discouraging. Woodruff et al. (1967) collected 23 patients treated with mercaptopurine; there were two responses. Talley (1973) saw no responses in 11 patients who received hydroxyurea. The response rate to hydroxyurea reported by Carter and Wasserman (7 of 25 patients or 28%) has not been found in other series. The lipid-soluble folate antagonist metoprine has produced tumor regression in 2 of 7 patients with renal cancer (Price et al. 1975; Currie et al. 1979) and one response lasted over a year. The apparent uselessness of other antimetabolites in renal cancer suggests that metoprine, with its lipid solubility and transport-independent cellular uptake, merits further study because these characteristics may confer therapeutic activity.

Vegetable Alkaloids

The report by Rhamey (Prout 1973) that 24 out of 75 patients (32%) treated with vinblastine showed objective regression of renal carcinoma has not been supported by others. Talley (1973) reported two regressions in 15 patients. Hrushesky (1977) from a literature review of 135 patients concluded that the response rate with vinblastine was 25%, but Carter and Wasserman's finding of 8% (1975) seems more credible. The related alkaloid vincristine has received inadequate study as a single agent and is invaluable when included in combined therapies. Epipodophyllotoxin (VP16-213) produced dramatic regression of pulmonary metastases of renal carcinoma in one of our patients, but in a systematic study by the Eastern Cooperative Oncology Group (Hahn 1977), the agent proved valueless.

Miscellaneous Agents

Cisplatin (cis-platinum diamminedichloride) was administered to 32 patients with metastatic kidney cancer by Rodriguez and Johnson (1978). In 23 evaluable patients there was one instance of minor tumor regression and in seven patients there was apparent stabilization of disease for 3–7 months. It was concluded that the therapeutic value of cisplatin is negligible when used a single agent in this disease. Talley (1973) treated 15 patients with antitumor antibiotics (actinomycin D, mithramycin, doxorubicin) with no responses; he found in the literature 23 patients treated with these agents with a single reported response. The Eastern Cooperative Oncology Group's study determined that galactitol is without useful activity in renal cancer (Hahn 1977).

Summary

A recent literature survey and review by Luderer et al. (1978) confirms the impression that the overall results of single-agent chemotherapy in carcinoma of the kidney are discouraging (Table 2.1). However, the number of properly controlled studies performed is inadequate and for many drugs the evidence that they are inactive is no more convincing than the evidence that some other drugs possess clinically useful activity. Only a few conclusions seem justified:
    1) the alkylating agents have no real value;
    2) the nitrosoureas appear to have minimal value in large series;
    3) antimetabolite drugs so far have not been shown to be useful;
    4) of the vegetable alkaloids, vinblastine has a reported response rate varying from 8% to 32%: the reasons for this disparity are unclear and more careful study is required;
    5) insofar as they have been assessed, cisplatin and the most potent antitumor antibiotics appear to be valueless.
It must be pointed out that as a result of the above findings, carcinoma of the kidney is an excellent tumor for well-designed prospective studies, including placebo studies, since there is no convincing evidence that any meaningful therapy has been identified. In this situation, evaluation of investigational drugs in formal trials is not only ethically permissible but ethically obligatory.

Table 2.1. Objective responses of carcinoma of the kidney to single chemotherapeutic agents. (Modified from Luderer et al. 1978)

Drug	No. of patients	Objective responses	
		Number	Percentage
Alkylating agents			
Cyclophosphamide	62	4	6
Chlorambucil	24	4	16
Mitomycin C	23	3	13
Miscellaneous	30	4	13
Nitrosoureas			
Lomustine (CCNU)	59	4	7
Semustine (MeCCNU)	21	0	0
Antimetabolites			
5-Fluorouracil	93	7	7.5
Mercaptopurine	29	2	7
Hydroxyurea	25	7	28[a]
Vegetable alkaloids			
Vinblastine	42	3	7
Vincristine	22	2	9
Miscellaneous			
Cisplatin	32	0	0
Bleomycin	26	3	11
Various antibiotics (doxorubicin, mithramycin, actinomycin D)	38	1	2.6

[a] This figure has not been confirmed by other investigators and is widely disbelieved by practising oncologists.

Multiple-Agent Chemotherapy

The principles of multiple-agent chemotherapy require the identification of single agents of proved activity, with differing mechanisms of action, and with toxic effects which do not completely overlap, so that the drugs may be used together in effective doses without prohibitive toxicity. In renal carcinoma, it is clear that the first prerequisite has not been met: better studies of single agents are needed before a rational combined drug therapy is essayed. Combining several drugs of negligible or nonexistent activity into a toxic regimen is most unlikely to produce satisfactory results. Nevertheless, multiple-agent cytotoxic chemotherapy currently is under active study in renal cancer.

Lokich and Harrison (1975) treated seven patients with combinations of up to five potent cytotoxic agents and saw no objective responses. Davis and Manalo (1978) treated 29 patients with a combination of lomustine and vinblastine and reported seven responses (24%). It is particularly interesting that two patients achieved a complete remission of 19+ and 24 months. No firm conclusion can of course be based on this small series. Luderer et al. (1978) collected from the literature 30 patients treated with a total of four multiple-drug regimens, with four objective responses (13%); one response was seen with each regimen. Again, no conclusion can be drawn from such data. Australian workers have used a combination of vinblastine, methotrexate, and bleomycin in 28 patients with metastatic renal cancer; half the patients also received tamoxifen (Levi et al. 1980). Five patients in each group (36%) had a partial response to this therapy and survival was prolonged in those who achieved partial response. This small study is promising but requires enlargement and confirmation.

Adjuvant Chemotherapy

The poor results of surgery in renal cancer (p. 10) indicate that occult metastatic disease is common at the time of operation. Promising, though as yet inconclusive, evidence that adjuvant chemotherapy may increase the cure rate in cancer of the breast (Bonadonna et al. 1976) has prompted studies of chemotherapy as an adjuvant to apparently complete surgical removal in other neoplasms where the surgical cure rate is poor — e.g. gastrointestional cancers and malignant melanoma.

It is debatable whether studies of adjuvant chemotherapy are yet appropriate in renal cancer. While it is true that the development of metastases after apparent surgical cure is common, the other prerequisite for adjuvant chemotherapy — possession of a regimen of known and high efficacy in established metastatic disease — has not been met in renal cancer as it has in breast cancer. Thus, the choice of an adjuvant regimen is certain to be ill-informed and very likely to be incorrect. This is exemplified by an uncontrolled study of adjuvant bleomycin and lomustine (CCNU) in 16 patients with stage 2 and stage 3 renal cancer who underwent potentially curative resection (Miller and Blom 1980). The inclusion of stage 2 patients is questionable, as their liability to metastatic disease is not demonstrably greater than for patients with stage 1 disease. The disease-free survival of 11 patients (69%) for a median of 3.7 years is not better than might be expected from surgical treatment alone, and two patients died from pulmonary toxicity attributable to bleomycin. If there is doubt as to the wisdom of initiating a formal trial of adjuvant chemotherapy in carcinoma of the kidney, there can be no doubt that the administration of adjuvant chemotherapy after surgery, outside the setting of an organized study, is at present without justification.

Immunotherapy

Although it has passed into common use, there are two objections to the term 'immunotherapy'. First, it has yet to be shown that it is therapeutic, and secondly, there is no good evidence in man that its mechanism of action (if it has any action) is immunological in nature. It might also be observed that in any disease, the tendency to employ immunotherapy is inversely proportional to the efficacy of the available chemotherapy. The occasional observation of spontaneous regressions of renal cancer raises the possibility that this tumor may sometimes be susceptible to a body defense mechanism which in turn might be an immunological one. The absence of any chemotherapy which inspires therapeutic enthusiasm makes it easier to study immunotherapy in this disease, since it does not involve denying the patient some established therapy of known value. It is doubtful whether this constitutes sufficient justification, especially if trials of immunotherapy are not accompanied by thorough evaluation of the immunological changes which accompany its administration.

Faulconer et al. (1978) have demonstrated possible tumor-associated antigens in human renal carcinoma. Cell-mediated immunity to these antigens was demonstrated in 63% of patients with renal cancer; normal renal tissue did not elicit an immune response. Reactivity to tumor-associated antigens was lost in patients who had had apparent surgical cure and persisted in patients with known metastases if they had not received cytotoxic agents. Antibodies to renal carcinoma were demonstrated by Ramming et al. (1977). These antibodies were present in patients with early metastatic disease and were unchanged so long as the disease was stable; antibody titers fell with disease progression. Antibody activity was absent in patients after apparent surgical cure and in patients with advanced metastatic disease. If confirmed, these observations would suggest that immune responses are mounted against renal cancer and decline if the tumor is removed. The immune response may hold metastatic disease in check and its failure may allow disease progression. The alternative hypothesis – that changes in immune status are a result, not a determinant, of tumor progression — cannot at present be disproved. Attempts to augment the immune response to renal cancer might have therapeutic potential. The recent demonstration (Ramming et al. 1979) that RNA from sheep immunized with human renal carcinoma elicits in rabbits antibody activity against a tumor-associated antigen not present in normal human renal tissue suggests the possibility of a specific immunotherapy which might be tested in patients. The theoretical risk of tumor enhancement by antibody seems not very great, since in man the progression of metastatic renal cancer seems to be accompanied by declining, rather than increasing, antibody activity.

Studies of human fibroblast leukocyte interferon in malignant disease are in an early stage; although not clinically useful, the interferons are of absorbing interest. In a preliminary report (McPherson and Tan 1979) four patients with renal cancer showed stable disease while receiving interferon; their disease progressed when treatment was discontinued. In a recent study (Bukowski et al. 1979) 31 patients with metastatic renal cancer received either lymphocyte transfer factor (TF), or TF with BCG vaccine, or (TF + BCG + lomustine + megestrol). Eight responses, including two complete remissions, were observed: three responses occurred in the non-chemotherapy groups. It may be significant that 6 of the 8 responses occurred in pulmonary sites: Luderer et al. (1978) have observed that the lung is the commonest site of response of renal cancer to cytotoxic drugs and hormones — and also the commonest site for spontaneous regression of tumor.

Prager et al. (1980) have treated 11 patients with autologous renal cancer cells complexed with a macrophage activating compound. Metastatic disease disappeared in two patients and was stable for more than 6 months in three patients. Circulating immunosuppressant substances were serially studied in eight patients, and there appeared to be some correlation between absence of immune suppressant activity in the serum and a favorable response to the immune stimulation. Unfortunately, parallel studies in control patients apparently were not done.

Obviously the evidence is inadequate for any verdict on the efficacy or otherwise of immunological manoeuvers in metastatic renal carcinoma. There are sufficient data to warrant further carefully controlled studies, which should include a placebo group or a no-therapy group. It seems inadvisable to confuse a difficult issue by combining immunological manipulation with cytotoxic drug therapy; unfortunately this has already begun (see p. 20, Multimodality Approaches to Renal Carcinoma).

Hormonal Manipulations

One basis for hormonal therapy lies in the observation that stilbestrol pellets implanted subcutaneously in male golden hamsters gave rise to adenomas and carcinomas of the kidney (Kirkman 1959). Removal of the pellets halted tumor growth, and administration of testosterone or progesterone with the stilbestrol inhibited tumor growth. Female hamsters and castrated males did not develop tumors when given stilbestrol implants. These observations suggested that both the genesis and the progression of renal cancers could be affected by disturbances of the hormonal milieu. It seems unlikely that androgens per se have a strong protective effect, since the incidence of renal cancer in men is twice that in women. Nor is it likely that physiological amounts of estrogens have a deleterious effect, for survival with renal cancer is not noticeably worse in women compared with men. The experimental observations were sufficient to prompt clinical studies, which seemed at first to have positive results. Although these results now are seriously questioned, the tendency to use hormonal therapy persists, partly because, in comparison to cytotoxic therapy, it is innocuous, and no doubt partly because there is a dearth of other promising measures which might be tried.

Progestational Agents

Samuels et al. (1968) treated 23 patients with metastatic renal cancer with medroxy-progesterone acetate; three patients (13% of the patients or 19% of the 16 patients who received the drug parenterally) showed an objective response. Wagle and Murphy (1971) reported six partial responses in 35 patients treated with parenteral medroxyprogesterone (17%); the duration of response varied from 3 to 31 months. Bloom (1973) collected from the literature 192 patients treated with progestogens or androgens and added 80 cases of his own: he found an overall objective response rate of 15%, with a range from 6% to 33%. In his own 80 patients, after excluding 20 who died within 6 weeks of beginning therapy, the response rate was 11/41 (27%) for men and 2/19 (10%) for women; 12 of the 13 responses were to medroxyprogesterone and one to testosterone. The responses usually were incomplete and of limited duration.

In his own patients, Bloom found 'subjective improvement' in 55%: the significance of this is unknown since there was no placebo-treated group. Papac et al. (1977) saw no objective responses in 12 patients treated with medroxyprogesterone.

The most comprehensive survey is that of Luderer et al. (1978). They collected results on 356 patients with renal carcinoma who were treated with a variety of progestational agents and recorded 30 responses (8%). It seems probable that spontaneous regression of renal cancer may occur in as few as 0.3% of cases (Bloom 1973) so it is likely that progestogens do indeed have some antitumor effect. Whether they prolong life, or improve it beyond the effect that might be expected from a placebo, is still uncertain. A more critical approach to hormonal therapy in renal cancer is reflected in the observation that, whereas the apparent response rate with hormones was 17% in 228 patients reported between 1967 and 1971, it was only 2% for 415 patients reported between 1971 and 1976 (Hrushesky 1977). The recent Eastern Cooperative Oncology Group study of megestrol (Hahn 1977) found no evidence that this progestational agent has any value.

Androgens

Androgenic hormones appear to be even less effective than progestational agents in metastatic renal carcinoma. Wagle and Murphy (1971) reported two objective responses in 27 patients (7.4%); one of these was a complete remission lasting 45 months. Bloom (1973) recorded only one response to testosterone in approximately 68 patients who failed to respond to medroxyprogesterone. Luderer et al. (1978) collected from the literature 188 patients treated with a variety of androgens: there were five objective responses (3%).

Androgens may be administered to cancer patients for their beneficial effect upon erythropoiesis and upon catabolism (Spiers and Allar 1979) and this may justify their use in selected patients with renal cancer, but it appears that the chance of securing objective regression of disease is remote.

Combined Hormonal Therapy

Agents which have dubious efficacy but do not possess additive toxicity are apt to be given in combination, perhaps with more optimism than science. A total of 48 patients treated with a combination of an androgen and a progestogen showed four objective responses (8.3%), which is no better than progestational agents alone (Luderer et al. 1978).

Hormone Antagonists

The antiestrogenic compound tamoxifen has undergone preliminary evaluation in renal cancer. Glick et al. (1979) saw no regression of tumor in 12 patients. They reported disease stabilization in two patients, which means little in a tumor as capricious as renal carcinoma. In a Southwest Oncology Group study (Al-Sarraf 1979) 49 patients received tamoxifen. There were two partial remissions (4%). Fourteen patients (28%) were stated to have 'improvement' or 'disease stabilization'. The author's conclusion that tamoxifen is active in renal cancer is debatable, and the suggestion that this agent now be included in multiple-drug regimens seems premature. A trial of tamoxifen in high dose (100 mg/m²/day) has begun, the rationale for these large doses being the known low affinity of the hormone receptors in renal tumor tissue (Papac et al. 1980, and also see below).

Hormone Receptors in Renal Cancer Tissue

Studies of hormone receptors have proved of clinical discriminant value in breast cancer and potentially might be of value in the management of patients with renal cancer. Concolino et al. (1978) studied cytosol estrogen and progesterone receptors in 23 renal cancers: 14 tumors (61%) were positive for each receptor. Unlike breast cancer tissue, the presence or absence of estrogen receptors had no correlation with that of progesterone receptors. Eighteen of these patients were treated with medroxyprogesterone acetate; there was no definite correlation between receptor status and response to therapy. Since 14 of 18 patients (78%) were considered to have a 'useful' response to hormonal therapy the clinical results clearly are not comparable with those from any other group.

In a recent study which compared specific steroid hormone binding in human renal carcinoma and normal kidney (Li et al. 1979) it appeared that renal tumor tissue contains less estrogen and glucocorticoid receptor than normal renal tissue, but similar amounts of progesterone receptor. Thus far, receptor studies have not been useful in dictating hormonal treatment for renal cancer, but the subject is still in its infancy. The apparent dissociation of estrogen receptor positivity and progesterone receptor positivity in renal tumors, in sharp contrast to the findings in breast cancer, raises the question of whether these receptor proteins have any biological role in renal tissue, or are in fact irrelevant to the behavior of renal tumors. A further possibility is that some 'receptors' are merely hormone-binding proteins which occur in the cytosol material, masquerade as receptor proteins in the assays currently used, but are not true receptors in the sense of mediating an effect of a steroid hormone upon the activities of a cell. Further basic research is needed to clarify these issues.

Summary

It appears that progestational agents are occasionally of benefit in renal cancer. Objective regression is seen in perhaps one patient in 12, but prolongation of life has not been proved. Subjective improvement certainly occurs, but the possibility that this is usually due to a placebo effect has not been tested. Androgens are not useful as antitumor agents but may benefit some patients because of their general anabolic effects. It is uncertain whether studies of hormone receptors in tumor tissue can improve the selection of patients for hormonal therapy. The results of hormonal therapy are at present so poor that trials of new cytotoxic drugs should take precedence over the use of progestogens in patients with good performance status and evaluable metastatic renal cancer.

Multimodality Approaches to Renal Carcinoma

The use of multimodality approaches, incorporating combinations of surgery, radiotherapy, chemotherapy, immunotherapy and hormonal manipulations, has greatly improved the management of certain cancers — for example Wilms' tumor and testicular cancer. Unfortunately, no profitable multimodality approach to renal cancer has been devised. The tumor is relatively radioresistant and in most instances is unresponsive to chemotherapy, so that it is difficult to plan a promising regimen. Preoperative or postoperative radiotherapy may lessen the incidence of local recurrences after surgery for a locally advanced primary tumor, but there is no evidence that the cure rate is enhanced.

Combinations of Cytotoxic Drugs and Hormones

Alberto and Senn (1974) treated 20 patients with the combination of a progestogen, an androgen, vinblastine and 5-fluorouracil: they reported no objective responses in these patients or in a further 40 patients who received either a progestogen or an androgen. Hahn et al. (1978) administered medroxyprogesterone and methyl-CCNU to 38 patients with metastatic renal cancer and observed one complete and three partial responses (11%). A further 38 patients were treated with medroxy-progesterone and vinblastine; there were three partial responses (8%). Performance status at entry to the trial, and a relatively long symptom-free interval between the initial surgery and the appearance of metastatic disease, were more significant prognostic factors than the type of therapy given. Katakkar and Franks (1978) reported a preliminary study in which eight patients received medroxyprogesterone with adriamycin, hydroxyurea, and vinblastine: there were three partial responses and one complete response. No conclusion can be drawn other than the necessity of extending this trial to include much larger numbers of patients.

Combinations of Cytotoxic Drugs, Hormones, and Immunotherapy

A combination of adriamycin, vincristine, medroxyprogesterone and BCG vaccine was administered to 14 patients by Ishmael et al. (1976). They reported one complete and four partial remissions (50% reduction in size of measurable lesions). The objective responses were short-lived, the mean duration of partial remission being 3 months. This series has since been enlarged (Ishmael et al. 1978) and 10 of 28 patients (36%) who received 6 weeks of treatment had an objective response. Most interesting was the experience of ten patients who had metastatic disease at the time of diagnosis. They underwent resection of the primary tumor followed by the combined regimen of cytotoxic, hormonal, and immunological therapy, and eight had an objective response (Ishmael et al. 1980, and p. 11, Surgery). Although the effect on survival so far is uncertain, these results certainly merit confirmatory studies with appropriate controls. Since about one-third of new patients with renal cancer have overt metastatic disease, there are numerous candidates for this seemingly promising approach.

Future Developments

From the foregoing review it is obvious that new developments and major improvements are needed in the management of metastatic carcinoma of the kidney. These may come from basic research or from experimental therapy.

Improved Hormonal Therapy

Refinements in the assay of steroidal receptors in renal cancer tissue, and an under-standing of their biological relevance (or lack of it) may facilitate the development of better hormonal approaches to renal tumors. Alternatively, receptor studies may only make it possible to identify the 8% of patients who may respond to a hormonal manipulation; this would reduce the number of futile trials of therapy but would not increase the absolute number of patients who experience some palliation of their disease. Certain phenomena regarding the responses of renal tumors to hormones (Luderer et al. 1978) do indeed suggest some sensitivity of this tumor to the endocrine milieu. Thus 81% of responses to progestogens were in men, and 72% of these were of pulmonary metastases. Of reported spontaneous regressions of renal cancer, 79% were in men and 95% are regressions of pulmonary deposits. The incidence of spontaneous regressions (0.3%–1%) is lower than that of response to progestogens (about 8%) but the underlying mechanism(s) may be similar. Further research, in man and in animal models, is warranted.

Immunological Approaches

Immunotherapy is a rational approach to malignant disease when it is studied with both appropriate randomized controls and laboratory surveillance of its effects. From an ethical standpoint, studies of this type are easiest to perform in diseases such as renal cancer where the 'orthodox' therapy is poor. Ramming and deKernion (1977) used RNA extracted from lymphoid organs of sheep immunized with human renal cancer tissue in 20 patients with metastatic renal cancer. They observed significantly increased survival in patients with lung metastases but RNA therapy did not influence survival of patients with metastases to other sites. Increased lympho-cyte-mediated cytotoxicity tests in RNA recipients were associated with an improved survival. The major defect of this interesting work is the use of historical controls. The occurrence of spontaneous remissions, the occasional regression of metastatic disease after the resection of a primary tumor, the hormonal responsiveness of pulmonary metastases, and the results of studies such as that described above, suggest than an immunological approach to renal cancer may eventually be profitable. The requirements for a successful trial include (a) large numbers of patients; (b) matched, randomized control subjects; (c) careful immunological surveillance during the trial. Unfortunately, the need for close laboratory monitoring restricts the numbers of institutions capable of mounting such trials and also makes the undertaking very costly.

Improved Chemotherapy

The continued development and testing of novel cytotoxic agents may eventually provide a drug with potent activity in carcinoma of the kidney. The problem with this approach is that it is slow, costly, and for the most part unpredictable. Such work must nevertheless continue because existing knowledge of cancer biology still does not permit the development of a rational therapy for renal cancer. The empirical approach, inefficient as it is, still merits clinical support.

Old drugs may still prove of value in renal cancer when administered in novel ways. The regional administration of mitomycin C encapsulated with methyl-cellulose (Kato et al. 1979) appears to have had beneficial effects in two patients, apparently converting one of them from inoperable to operable. Recent studies (Ghose et al. 1978) have shown that cytotoxic drugs can be linked to antibodies specific for renal cancer tissue: this approach deserves clinical study. The antitumor agent methylglyoxal-bis-guanylhydrazone (methyl-GAG), long neglected because of its prohibitive toxicity, has recently been found to possess an augmented therapeutic index when administered by a weekly, instead of a daily, schedule. In a preliminary report (Knight et al. 1979), three of four patients with metastatic renal cancer responded to methyl-GAG. Two further reports (Knight et al. 1980, Todd et al. 1980) describe a total of 32 evaluable patients who received weekly doses of methyl-GAG. Seven patients (22%) responded, with two complete and five partial remissions. Toxicity, particularly gastrointestinal disturbances, was significant but not life-threatening. Among the 18 patients evaluated in Boston, three of the four responses observed were regression of pulmonary metastases (Todd et al. 1980). Methyl-GAG appears to have definite, if limited, activity in carcinoma of the kidney.

As Carter and Wasserman (1975) pointed out, many drugs have had inadequate evaluation in renal cancer, and it is possible that agents effective in this tumor are already in our possession. Phase II studies of chemotherapy, unlike sophisticated studies of immunotherapy, can be conducted at many centers, and cooperative multicenter trials should continue.

The acridine derivative acridinylamino-methanesulfon-m-anisidine (mAMSA) is active in several tumors, including acute myeloid leukemia. Administration to 16 patients with stage 4 renal carcinoma resulted in no tumor regressions (Fuks et al. 1980). For unknown reasons, renal cancers are resistant to agents that attack preformed DNA, even though the agents shown to be ineffective (cyclophosphamide, adriamycin, nitrosoureas, cisplatinum, mAMSA) do not have identical mechanisms of action.

Temporary Nephrectomy

Prout (1973) drew attention to the fact that removal of a kidney and maintenance by perfusion in vitro for several hours before reimplantation is well within present technical capabilities. A patient with metastatic renal cancer might undergo removal of the primary tumor, temporary removal of the normal kidney, and be treated for several hours with one of the many potent nephrotoxic agents available. The kidney would be reimplanted after the drug had been neutralized by an antidote, detoxified by the liver, or removed by hemodialysis. The trouble with this approach is that there are many nephrotoxic substances to choose from – some also have hepatic or vestibular toxicity — and there is no guarantee that renal cancer will be susceptible to agents which poison normal tubular epithelium. There is an understandable hesitancy to perform major surgery for such problematical gains.

Studies of the Biology of Renal Carcinoma

Apart from the existence of animal models, human renal cancers can readily be grown in vitro. Detailed studies of the immunology, growth kinetics, and cell membrane biochemistry of these tumors may make possible rational chemical attack.

A recent report (Cohen et al. 1979) has shown an association between familial renal cancer and a constitutional chromosomal anomaly, a reciprocal translocation between chromosomes 3 and 8, designated t(3; 8) (p 14; q 24). This anomaly occurred in a family with ten cases of renal cancer in three generations; other hallmarks of familial cancer — early age of onset and 60% of tumors being bilateral — were also present. Present mapping of the affected chromosomes is very incomplete, but here is an obvious biological clue to the genesis of renal cancer and also, perhaps to ways in which a chemotherapeutic attack may be mounted.

A Policy for the Patient with Metastatic Renal Cancer

Renal cancer presents a challenge, but few rewards, to the chemotherapist. There is ample scope for research in this tumor, but our ability to effect major improvement in individual patients is severely limited. A treatment policy should avoid over-zealous therapy which may diminish the quality of a patient's life; equally it should avoid therapeutic nihilism and the failure to investigate new treatments. The practising urologist and medical oncologist have the dual aims of offering to each patient the best palliation while at the same time advancing our knowledge of renal cancer.

The newly diagnosed patient with renal cancer and overt metastases, whose general physical condition is good, may be considered for a vigorous therapeutic approach. This may include resection of the primary tumor, removal of large accessible metastases, and combined cytotoxic, hormonal, and immunological therapy (Ishmael et al. 1978). This is best done in the setting of a formal clinical trial, but may also be considered on an ad hoc basis for the young and otherwise robust patient with renal carcinoma.

Many patients are quite unsuitable, for a variety of medical and psychological reasons, for such an aggressive approach. A trial of chemotherapy may however be appropriate. If possible, such patients should be entered into a Phase II drug study, where they may benefit both from the agent under test and from the advantages of a carefully designed and tested protocol. There is a great need for more data on the responsiveness of renal tumors to a variety of new and old cytotoxic drugs.

If the possibility does not exist for entering the patient into a formal trial, drug therapy may be deferred until progression of disease has been documented, since metastatic disease may remain apparently stationary for weeks or months without therapeutic intervention and causing no symptoms. When advancing and/or symptomatic disease is present, a trial of vinblastine is justifiable in most patients. Although there is dissension about the objective response rate with vinblastine, it has the advantages of only moderate toxicity and a well-established dose schedule. It may be combined with a progestational agent — for example weekly intramuscular medroxyprogesterone — which adds very little in the way of toxicity.

The old or frail patient, and those with very advanced disease, may be candidates only for a trial of a progestational agent. This offers a low response rate but also a low toxicity. There is usually psychological benefit for the patient (and his physician) in the knowledge that some type of treatment is being offered. Certainly there is no place for aggressive cytotoxic drug therapy in the patient with a high tumor burden and in poor general condition, particularly if hepatic, renal, or bone marrow function are already compromised. In this setting one can virtually guarantee severe toxicity and there is no prospect of a clinically useful tumor response.

Because the disease may be slowly progressive, or progress intermittently, the palliative care of patients with metastatic renal cancer may be long-drawn-out. Analgesic and psychotropic drugs, radiotherapy, and orthopedic and neurosurgical measures, may all be required. Not infrequently, hospice-type care is indicated. The successful management of these unfortunate patients, who are often immobile and in pain from multiple skeletal metastases, requires therapeutic skill and personal compassion of a high order.

References

Alberto P, Senn HJ (1974) Hormonal therapy of renal carcinoma alone and in association with cytostatic drugs. Cancer 33: 1226–1229

Al-Sarraf M (1979) The clinical trial of tamoxifen in patients with advanced renal cell cancer. A Southwest Oncology Group study. Proc Am Soc Clin Oncol 20: 378, C-360

American Cancer Society (1973) Cancer facts and figures. New York: American Cancer Society

Bloom HJG (1973) Hormone-induced and spontaneous regression of metastatic renal cancer. Cancer 32: 1066–1071

Bonadonna G, Brusamolino E, Valagussa P, Rossi A, Brugnatelli L, Brambilla C, De Lena M, Tancini G, Bajetta E, Musumeci R, Veronesi U (1976) Combination chemotherapy as an adjuvant treatment in operable breast cancer. N Engl J Med 294: 405–410

Bukowski RM, Groppe C, Reimer R, Weick J, Hewlett JS (1979) Immunotherapy (IT) of metastatic renal cell carcinoma. Proc Am Soc Clin Oncol 20: 402, C-457

Carter RL (1968) The pathology of renal cancer. JAMA 204: 221–222

Carter SK, Wasserman TH (1975) The chemotherapy of urologic cancer. Cancer 36: 729–747

Cohen AJ, Li FP, Berg S, Marchetto DJ, Tsai S, Jacobs SC, Brown RS (1979) Hereditary renal-cell carcinoma associated with a chromosomal translocation. N Engl J Med 310: 592–595

Concolino G, Marocchi A, Conti C, Tenaglia R, Di Silverio F, Bracci U (1978) Human renal cell carcinoma as a hormone-dependent tumor. Cancer Res 38: 4340–4344

Currie VE, Kempin SJ, Sykes MP, Young CW (1979) Clinical studies of 2,4-diamino-5-(3'4'-dichlorophenyl)-6-methylpyrimidine (metoprine) with and without leucovorin. Proc Am Assoc Cancer Res 20: 112, 454

Davis TE, Manalo FB (1978) Combination chemotherapy of advanced renal cell cancer with CCNU and vinblastine. Proc Am Soc Clin Oncol 19: 316, C-39

Everson TC, Cole WH (1966) Spontaneous regression of cancer. Saunders, Philadelphia London

Faulconer RJ, Rosato FE, Wright GL, Schellhammer P (1978) Detection and isolation of antigens associated with renal cell carcinoma. Proc Am Soc Clin Oncol 19: 308, C-8

Fuks JZ, Van Echo DA, Aisner J, Kravitz S, Wiernik PH (1980) A Phase II trial of 4'-(9-acrindinyl-amino)-methanesulfon-m-anisidine (AMSA) in patients with renal cell carcinoma (RCC) and refractory small cell carcinoma of the lung (SCCL). Proc Am Soc Clin Oncol 21: 477, C-622

Ghose T, Tai J, Blair AH, Belitsky P, Aquino J, Norvell ST (1978) Antitumor antibodies as carriers of radionucleides and cytotoxic drugs. Proc Am Assoc Cancer Res 19: 236, 942

Glick J, Wein A, Negendank W, Harris D, Brodovsky H, Padavic K, Torri S (1979) Tamoxifen in metastatic prostate and renal cancer. Proc Am Soc Clin Oncol 20: 311, C-81

Grawitz P (1883) Die sogenannten Lipomas der Niere. Virchow Arch [Pathol Anat] 93: 39–63

Hahn RG (1977) Megace, VP-16, cytoxan and galactitol. Phase II treatment trials in advanced renal cell cancer. Proc Am Soc Clin Oncol 18: 332, C-262

Hahn RG, Temkin NR, Savlov ED, Perlia C, Wampler GL, Horton J, Marsh J, Carbone PP (1978) Phase II study of vinblastine, methyl-CCNU, and medroxyprogesterone in advanced renal cell cancer. Cancer Treat Rep 62: 1093–1095

Hrushesky WJ (1977) What's old and new in advanced renal cell carcinoma. Proc Am Soc Clin Oncol 18: 318, C-206

Ishmael DR, Bottomley R, Geyer J (1980) Effect of nephrectomy on eventual response to chemotherapy in renal cell carcinoma. Proc Am Soc Clin Oncol 21: 429, C-439

Ishmael DR, Bottomley RH, Hoge AF (1976) Treatment of renal cell adenocarcinoma (hypernephroma) with Depo-Provera and combination chemoimmunotherapy. Proc Am Soc Clin Oncol 17: 265, C-113

Ishmael DR, Burpo LJ, Bottomley RH (1978) Combined therapy of advanced hypernephroma with medroxyprogesterone, BCG, adriamycin and vincristine. Proc Am Soc Clin Oncol 19: 407, C-403

Katakkar SB, Franks CR (1978) Chemo-hormonal therapy for metastatic renal cell carcinoma with adriamycin, hydroxyurea, vinblastine, and medroxyprogesterone acetate. Cancer Treat Rep 62: 1379–1380

Kato T, Nemoto R, Mori H, Kumagai I (1979) Microencapsulated mitomycin-C therapy in renal cell carcinoma. Lancet II: 479–480

Kirkman H (1959) Estrogen-induced tumors of the kidney in the Syrian hamster. Natl Cancer Inst Mongr 1: 1–37

Kirulata G, Morales A, Lott S (1975) Response of renal adenocarcinoma to cyclophosphamide. Urology 6: 557–558

Knight WA, Livingston RB, Fabian C, Costanzi J (1979) Methyl-glyoxal bis-guanylhydrazone (methyl-GAG, MGBG) in advanced human malignancy. Proc Am Soc Clin Oncol 20: 319, C-115

Knight WA, Livingston RB, Fabian C, Costanzi J (1980) Methyl-glyoxal bis-guanulhydrazone (methyl-GAG, MGBG) in advanced renal carcinoma. Proc Am Soc Clin Oncol 21: 367, C-190

Kradjian JM, Bennington JL (1964) Renal carcinoma recurrent 31 years after nephrectomy. Arch Surg 90: 192–195

Levi JA, Dalley D, Aroney R (1980) A comparative trial of the combination vinblastine (V), methotrexate (A) and bleomycin (B) with and without tamoxifen (T) for metastatic renal cell carcinoma (RCC). Proc Am Soc Clin Oncol 21: 426, C-425

Li JJ, Li SA, Gonzales R (1979) Specific hormone binding in human renal carcinoma and kidney. Proc Am Assoc Cancer Res 20: 273, 1107

Lokich JL, Harrison JH (1975) Renal cell carcinoma: natural history and chemotherapeutic experience. J Urol 114: 371–374

Luderer RC, Opipari MI, Perrotta AL (1978) Treatment of metastatic renal cell carcinoma: Review of experience and world literature. Journal of the American Osteopathic Association 77: 590–603

McPherson TA, Tan YH (1979) Phase I study of human fibroblast interferon (FI) in human malignancy. Proc Am Soc Clin Oncol 20: 378, C-361

Middleton RG (1967) Surgery for metastatic renal cell carcinoma. J Urol 97: 973–977

Miller CF, Blom J (1980) Adjuvant chemotherapy of renal cell carcinoma using a combination of bleomycin (BLM) and lomustine (CCNU). Proc Am Soc Clin Oncol 21: 362, C-171

Mittelman A, Albert DJ, Murphy GP (1973) Lomustine treatment of metastatic renal cell carcinoma. JAMA 225: 32–35

Papac R, Luikhart S, Kirkwood J (1980) High-dose tamoxifen in patients with advanced renal cell cancer and malignant melanoma. Proc Am Soc Clin Oncol 21: 358, C-155

Papac RJ, Ross AS, Levy A (1977) Renal cell carcinoma: analysis of 31 cases with assessment of endocrine therapy. Am J Med Sci 274: 281–289

Prager MD, Peters PC, Baechtel FS, Brown G (1980) Specific immunotherapy of metastatic human renal cell carcinoma: preliminary results. Proc Am Assoc Cancer Res 21: 213, 856

Price LA, Goldie JH, Hill BT (1975) Methodichlorophen as anti-tumour drug. Br Med J i: 20–21

Prout GR (1973) The kidney and ureter. In: Holland JF, Frei E (eds) Cancer medicine. Lea & Febiger, Philadelphia, pp 1655–1669

Ramming KP, deKernion JB (1977) Immune RNA therapy for renal cell carcinoma: Survival and immunologic monitoring. Ann Surg 186: 459–466

Ramming KP, Gupta RK, deKernion JB (1977) Detection of antibodies to tumor associated antigens in patients with hypernephroma. Proc Amer Soc Clin Oncol 18: 319, C-211

Ramming KP, Gupta RK, deKernion JB (1979) Induction of antibody to human renal cell cancer in vivo by injections of xenogeneic immune RNA. Proc Am Assoc Cancer Res 20: 215, 872

Robson CJ, Churchill BM, Anderson W (1969) The results of radical nephrectomy for renal cell carcinoma. J Urol 101: 297–301

Rodriguez LH, Johnson DE (1978) Clinical trial of cisplatinum (NSC 119875) in metastatic renal cell carcinoma. Urology 11: 344–346

Samuels ML, Sullivan P, Howe CD (1968) Medroxyprogesterone acetate in the treatment of renal cell carcinoma (hypernephroma). Cancer 22: 525–532

Spiers ASD, Allar M (1979) Beneficial effects of concurrent androgen treatment during cytotoxic chemotherapy. Proc Am Soc Clin Oncol 20: 295, C-8

Talley RW (1973) Chemotherapy of adenocarcinoma of the kidney. Cancer 32: 1062–1065

Todd RF, Garnick MB, Canellos GP (1980) Chemotherapy of advanced renal adenocarcinoma with methyl-glyoxal-bis-guanylhydrazone (methyl-GAG). Proc Am Soc Clin Oncol 21: 340, C-85

Wagle DG, Murphy GP (1971) Hormonal therapy in advanced renal cell carcinoma. Cancer 28: 318–321

Wajsman Z, Beckley S, Madajewucz S, Dragone N (1980) High-dose cyclophosphamide (CPM) in metastatic renal cell cancer. Proc Am Soc Clin Oncol 21: 423, C-413

Woodruff MW, Wagle D, Gailani SD, Jones R (1967) The current status of chemotherapy for advanced renal carcinoma. J Urol 97: 611–618

Chapter 3

The Management of Wilms' Tumor

J. E. Champion, J. Wilimas and A. P. M. Kumar

Introduction

The history of Wilms' tumor is one of the success stories of pediatric oncology and serves as a model for a multispecialty approach to childhood cancer. The foundation of this approach includes a surgical pathologic staging system that reflects prognosis and therefore defines therapy. A multidisciplinary approach which includes pediatric and urological surgeons, pathologists, radiotherapists and pediatric oncologists can provide treatment programs which utilize the benefits of surgery, radiation therapy and multiagent chemotherapy. Increasing concerns about long-term complications of therapy in view of ever-increasing survival has underlined the need for careful reappraisal of the benefits and risks of each modality.

Reviews of surgical therapy show a 15%–30% cure rate in patients undergoing nephrectomy alone (Abeshouse 1957; Harvey 1950; Klapproth 1959; Scott 1956). The addition of radiotherapy increased the overall survival with cure rates as high as 46% (Gross and Neuhauser 1950). Farber's work with dactinomycin (Farber et al. 1960) reported in 1960 and Sutow's report on vincristine in 1965 (Sutow 1965), showed increased survival even among patients with metastatic disease. Recent results of multimodal therapy show that patients presenting without extra-abdominal metastases at diagnosis have a 90% 2-year survival (National Wilms' Tumor Study: unpublished results). Due to this improvement in survival, the aim of therapy becomes survival without excessive morbidity or long-term complications.

Incidence

The incidence of Wilms' tumor is similar for all races at 5.0–7.8 per million children per year under the age of 15 years (Marsden and Steward 1968; Young and Miller 1975). Wilms' tumor accounts for about 6% of all pediatric malignancies and 11.1% of all non-lymphomatous solid tumors (Marsden and Steward 1968; Young and Miller 1975). There appears to be no sex predilection. Cumulative data reveal a predominance of left-sided tumors. The tumor is bilateral at diagnosis in 4.7% of patients (Table 3.1). The peak age at diagnosis is between 1 and 3 years, with 90% of all cases diagnosed in patients less than 7 years of age. The experience of the authors is very similar to that reported for Sutow's 826 cases (Sutow et al. 1977) (Table 3.2).

Table 3.1. Clinical features of Wilms' tumor

	Sex		1° Site		Laterality		
	Male	Female	Left	Right	Unilateral	Bilateral	% Bilateral
Literature	1087[a]	1123[a]	551[b]	448[b]	3663[c]	172[c]	4.5%
SJCRH	78	72	62	74	136	14	9.3%
Total	1165	1195	613	522	3799	186	4.7%
Ratio	0.97:1		1.17:1		20.4:1		

[a] References: Baert et al. 1966; Bond 1975; Cassady et al. 1977; Currie et al. 1973; Everson and Fraumeni 1975; Garcia et al. 1963; Green and Jaffe 1978; Knudson and Strong 1972; Morris Jones et al. 1978; Pendergrass 1976; Perez et al. 1973; Platt and Linden 1964; Young and Miller 1975.
[b] References: Aron 1974; Baert et al. 1966; Cassady et al. 1977; Currie et al. 1973; Garcia et al. 1963; Ledlie et al. 1970; Lennox et al. 1979; Morris Jones et al. 1978.
[c] References in [b] and: Bishop et al. 1977; Bond 1975; Knudson and Strong 1972; Lemerle et al. 1976a; Ragab et al. 1972.
SJCRH — St. Jude Children's Research Hospital, Memphis, Tennessee.

Table 3.2. Age incidence of Wilms' tumor

Age	SJCRH	% of Total	Cumulative %	Sutow et al. (1977) Cumulative %
0–1	19	12.7	12.7	12.8
1–2	31	20.7	33.3	31.2
2–3	23	15.3	48.7	49.2
3–4	29	19.3	68.0	65.7
4–5	13	8.7	76.7	77.1
5–6	10	6.7	83.3	85.3
6–7	12	8.0	91.3	90.9
7–8	4	2.7	94.0	93.7
>8	9	6.0	100.0	100.0
		100.0		

SJCRH — St. Jude Children's Research Hospital, Memphis, Tennessee.

Genetics and Associated Anomalies

An embryonic origin of Wilms' tumor, or nephroblastoma, was suggested by Wilms (1899). This is supported by its occurrence in early childhood, by its association with congenital anomalies and by the finding of a precursor benign lesion that can develop into Wilms' tumor. A disorder in the embryogenesis of the metanephric ridge is associated with a subsequent increased susceptibility to malignancy of this structure. Wilms' tumor has been observed in the neonate or fetus as well as the young infant (Klapproth 1959; Richmond and Dougall 1970). Neonatal Wilms' tumor must be distinguished from benign tumors which include mesoblastic nephroma, nodular renal blastema, and nephroblastomatosis (Richmond and Dougall 1970; Shanklin and Sotelo-Avila 1969). In situ nephroblastoma has been reported in 0.42% of infant autopsies less than 4 months of age (Shanklin and Sotelo-Avila 1969). Nodular renal blastema, a benign cortical collection of primitive embryonic renal cells, is associated with development of Wilms' tumor and with a chromosomal abnormality, trisomy 18 (Bove et al. 1969; Rous et al. 1976).

A genetic influence on the development of Wilms' tumor has been further supported by the unusual feature of tumor involvement of both kidneys simultaneously or sequentially. Bilateral Wilms' tumor occurs in a younger age group than unilateral tumor with a mean age at diagnosis of 2 years (Cochran and Froggart 1967). Furthermore, reports of familial occurrence of Wilms' tumor with an increased incidence of bilaterality in these families led Knudson to postulate a two-mutational model for Wilms' tumor similar to that proposed for retinoblastoma (Knudson and Strong 1972). Knudson's hypothesis requires two mutations in order for familial or bilateral Wilms' tumor to occur. The first may be prezygotic (inherited) or postzygotic (after conception) with the second mutation always postzygotic. From the available data, Knudson suggested the initial mutation was inherited in 38% of Wilms' tumor patients. Of those children who inherit this mutation from a parent, 37% will not develop a tumor, 48% will have a unilateral lesion and 15% will develop bilateral involvement (Knudson and Strong 1972). Although no chromosomal abnormalities have been consistently associated with Wilms' tumor, patients with trisomy 18 and nodular renal blastema (Bove et al. 1969) or aniridia with deletion of the short arm of chromosome 11(11p$-$) (Riccardi et al. 1978) have been noted to have an increased incidence of Wilms' tumor.

Three major anomalies have been associated with Wilms' tumor. Green and Jaffe (1978) reviewed reports on 1570 patients with Wilms' tumor from four investigators (Ledlie et al. 1970; Lemerle et al. 1976a; Miller et al. 1964; Pendergrass 1976). They found 17 patients (1.08%) with aniridia, 28 patients (1.78%) with hemihypertrophy, and 83 patients (5.28%) with a variety of genito-urinary anomalies. Fraumeni and Glass (1968) noted a 25% (7/28) frequency of Wilms' tumor in patients admitted for sporadic and familial aniridia. Six of the seven cases demonstrated the sporadic form of aniridia.

Hemihypertrophy, usually idiopathic, may occur isolateral or contralateral to the tumor site and may be present at diagnosis of Wilms' tumor or emerge later (Fraumeni et al. 1967). Another syndrome associated with tissue overgrowth, the Beckwith-Wiedemann syndrome (omphalocele, macroglossia and gigantism), is associated with a 10% probability of neoplasia. In one report, Wilms' tumor accounted for 6 of the 14 neoplasms followed in frequency by adrenal carcinoma and hepatoblastoma (Sotelo-Avila and Gooch 1976).

Genito-urinary anomalies associated with Wilms' tumor include ectopic and solitary kidneys, horseshoe kidneys, ureteric duplications, hypospadias, and cryptorchidism (Green and Jaffe 1978, Pendergrass 1976). The association of Wilms' tumor with pseudohermaphroditism and nephrotic syndrome is recorded in sporadic reports (Barakat et al. 1974; Lines 1968; Spear et al. 1971). Perlman noted a combination of genito-urinary anomalies, renal hamartomas, fetal gigantism and nephroblastomatosis associated with Wilms' tumor (Perlman et al. 1975).

Clinical Presentation

Clinical presentations of children with Wilms' tumor include abdominal swelling and palpable mass (84%), abdominal pain (35%–40%), fever (23%), hematuria (12%–24%), weight loss, anorexia, pallor, and nausea and vomiting (Aron 1974; Baert et al. 1966; Green and Jaffe 1978); Lemerle et al. 1976a; Perez et al. 1973). Other less common presenting features that initially do not suggest tumor are inguinal hernia and enlarged testes (Cassady et al. 1973), congestive heart failure (Sanyal et al. 1976), and symptomatic pleural effusions (Betkerur and Lanzkowsky

1977; Jaffe et al. 1973). Twelve percent of patients with Wilms' tumors may present with symptoms of an acute intra-abdominal emergency (Lemerle et al. 1976a).

The association of hypertension with Wilms' tumor was first reported in 1938 (Bradley and Pincoffs 1938). Later Sukarochana et al. (1972) reported a 63% occurrence of systolic or systolic-diastolic hypertension in 46 patients studied. Increased serum renin levels were noted in several reports (Ganguly et al. 1973; Sukarochana et al. 1972). Suggested etiologies of the increased renin production include excessive secretion by the tumor cells (Ganguly et al. 1973) or renal ischemia caused by tumor compression of renal arteries (Sukarochana et al. 1972). Relief of hypertension occurs 2–3 weeks after surgical resection. The occurrence of hypertension has had no correlation with duration of survival (Marsden and Steward 1968; Sukarochana et al. 1972).

A complete history should note onset and duration of any abdominal complaints, hematuria, vomiting, fever, recent infection or trauma. Maternal prenatal history, neonatal problems as well as family history of neoplasia or physical abnormalities are necessary for a complete evaluation. Although the initial physical examination may center around palpation and inspection of the abdominal mass, special attention should be given to blood pressure, eyes (aniridia), facial and extremity symmetry (hemihypertrophy) and external genitalia (hypospadias, hernia, cryptorchidism). The pulmonary and cardiac examination can detect effusions, murmurs or symptoms of heart failure that might signify extension of Wilms' tumor into the chest structures causing future problems in surgery. Right-sided Wilms' tumor should be distinguished from hepatomegaly (congestive heart failure, infiltrative diseases of the liver or malignancies, i.e., leukemia, neuroblastoma and hepatoblastoma). The examining physician should be alerted to secondary complications by such nonspecific features as pallor indicating anemia, fever from infection or tumor necrosis, edema suggesting nephrotic syndrome, and cardiorespiratory distress reflecting congestive heart failure, pulmonary infiltrate or pleural effusion.

When all laboratory and radiographic evidence for an intrarenal tumor is consistent with Wilms' tumor, there still exists an 8% incidence of false diagnosis on subsequent surgery and pathologic evaluation (D'Angio et al. 1976; Green and Jaffe 1978; Lemerle et al. 1976b). Neuroblastoma accounts for one-third of all the incorrect preoperative diagnoses (Green and Jaffe 1978).

Laboratory investigation should include a full blood count, evaluation of liver and renal function, serum uric acid and urinalysis. A urine spot test for catecholamines may be helpful in distinguishing neuroblastoma from Wilms' tumor (Table 3.3). Radiographic evaluation should include an initial plain abdominal X-ray. Punctate

Table 3.3.   Current recommended and optional tests in evaluation of intrarenal abdominal tumor

Blood studies	Hemoglobin, leukocyte count with differential, platelet count and reticulocyte count, blood urea nitrogen, creatinine, SGOT, SGPT, alkaline phosphatase, total protein, albumin, globulin, bilirubin, uric acid
Urine	Urinalysis, spot catecholamine-VMA
X-Rays	Plain film of the abdomen Intravenous urogram Chest X-ray including lateral Abdominal ultrasound with attention to the inferior vena cava [a]Liver spleen scan
Optional[a]	Inferior vena cavagram Bone scan, skeletal survey, bone marrow aspiration Chest and abdominal computerized tomography

[a] If indicated, generally postoperative.

calcifications can occur in Wilms' tumor at sites of hemorrhage, but are more frequently associated with neuroblastomas and teratomas. An intravenous urogram is generally the most helpful diagnostic tool. It distinguishes an intrarenal mass from an adrenal or perinephric mass that may displace normal kidney structure. Hydronephrosis and infantile polycystic kidneys are also distinguished by typical radiographic features. An intrarenal mass is more consistent with displacement, distortion or obliteration of renal calyceal structure. A routine chest X-ray evaluates the lungs for metastases.

Further evaluation by more sophisticated techniques requires a diagnostic imaging department experienced in ultrasonography, pediatric angiography, radionuclide scanning and computerized tomography. Benefits, risks, necessity and efficacy of these modalities are still being evaluated for diagnosis and staging of Wilms' tumor.

Ultrasonography of the renal fossa and abdomen can distinguish cystic from solid masses by the presence of multiple echogenic foci within the solid mass. Ultrasonography can also determine if the mass is intrarenal or extrarenal, by outlining the major fascial planes, the renal capsule and the calyces. Ultrasonography of the inferior vena cava and right atrium is a non-invasive presurgical test that can demonstrate tumor invasion. If positive, the ultrasonography should be followed by angiography and surgical exploration (Schullinger et al. 1977; Slovis et al. 1978).

Evaluation for distant metastases can be performed after initial resection of the primary tumor, since therapy for metastatic lesions is primarily nonsurgical. Nuclear scanning of the liver and spleen can identify tumor invasion or metastases. The diagnosis of hepatic metastasis is generally made at laparatomy and confirmed on pathologic review of a liver biopsy. If pathologic evaluation of the primary renal tumor demonstrates an abnormality associated with metastasis to bone, i.e., sarcomatous or anaplastic clear cell variant, then bone marrow aspiration and biopsy, technetium bone scan and skeletal survey are indicated.

A recent advance in diagnostic imaging, computerized tomography (CT) allows earlier detection of pulmonary and intra-abdominal metastases. Initial impressions suggest that CT could more accurately stage the patient and thereby influence selection of optimal therapy and affect overall survival. However, the current staging system was developed with conventional radiographic studies, and has effectively predicted the stage dependent prognosis. It remains to be determined if pulmonary lesions detected by CT but not by chest X-rays have the same prognostic significance as larger nodules. Our current approach is to obtain a baseline CT of the chest but not to change the staging of the patient and increase therapy and toxicity because of suspicious lesions seen on CT alone. This approach will change if analysis of the outcome of patients with only CT positive chest lesions demonstrates subsequent relapses in sites predicted by CT.

Abdominal CT of the infant or small child is complicated by the absence of the radiologist's standard reference, periaortic and perinephric fat. This study is performed postoperatively to evaluate its capability for detecting abdominal recurrence. For satisfactory CT the regular metal clips, previously used for marking surgical margins for radiotherapy, must be replaced by as few titanium clips as possible to reduce distortion artifact.

Surgical Approach

Surgery remains the mainstay of diagnosis and therapy for Wilms' tumor, but any surgical procedures beyond nephrectomy should be discussed with the radiotherapist and pediatric oncologist. A wide transabdominal approach is the standard recommendation because it allows examination of the entire abdomen, both kidneys, adrenals, liver and lymph nodes. With this approach massive lesions can be more easily removed without rupturing the tumor capsule. The flank approach for Wilms' tumor has become unacceptable due to the often large size of the tumor, the 8% incidence of false positive Wilms' tumor diagnosis, and the incidence of bilaterality that may be expressed as a small cortical tumor on the opposite kidney. A review of the effects on survival of a flank incision (Aron 1974) noted a 52% 2-year survival for patients who had flank incision compared to 67% for those patients who had transabdominal incisions.

After opening the peritoneum, the abdominal cavity should be examined for tumor spread and suspicious areas biopsied. Free peritoneal fluid or blood should be collected for cytology. After abdominal exploration, the peritoneum is incised lateral to the colon and the colon moved medially to expose the tumor, aorta and inferior vena cava. The vena cava is palpated for tumor thrombus and if present the thrombus is removed after the primary renal tumor is excised. The renal pedicle is isolated and tied, allowing an adequate length of renal vein, artery and ureter for pathologic evaluation of tumor invasion. The kidney and tumor are removed by blunt dissection with care that the capsule of the tumor is not disrupted. In order to remove the tumor in toto, any adherent perinephric fat, bowel or adrenal gland is excised. Examination of perihilar and para-aortic nodes is performed with excision of any suspicious or enlarged nodes. Total lymph node dissection probably is not necessary, since treatment is not changed if more than one node is positive for tumor. Chemotherapy and radiation can control any residual, non-enlarged, lymph nodes involved with tumor. Prolongation of anesthesia in order to perform an extensive multiple lymph node dissection is not justified in young infants and small children because these metastases generally are sensitive to therapy. The liver is inspected and any suspicious nodules are biopsied. The opposite kidney must be fully mobilized, and its entire posterior surface inspected. Any abnormality of the renal parenchyma is biopsied.

When complete resection is not possible, because the tumor has adhered to adjacent structures preventing any approach to the renal hilum or fossa, biopsy is followed by radiation and chemotherapy and a second surgical approach may become possible. Because this tumor is so responsive to radiotherapy and chemotherapy, extensive resection of bowel, muscle, liver or other organs currently is not recommended. Complete resection can be attempted with very large tumors if, despite massive size, the tumor remains encapsulated and is easily freed from other structures. Resection of metastatic lesions must be individualized in each case since most lesions are sensitive to chemotherapy and radiation.

Surgical-Pathologic Staging

The primary goal of any staging system is to identify patients who will have different chances of survival because of certain consistent prognostic features, and who thereby have a greater or lesser need for adjuvant therapy. The surgeon determines the clinical stage by observation during exploratory laparotomy while the pathologist confirms or amends those findings by histologic evaluation.

Outlined in Table 3.3 are the staging criteria found by the authors to be practical and valid. Basic features of the system identify stage I as localized, all tumor removed; stage II, microscopic residual tumor; stage III, more significant and possible gross residual tumor; stage IV, metastatic disease beyond the abdomen, stage V, the special circumstance of bilateral disease at diagnosis. Garcia et al. (1963)

identified weight of the tumor as a major prognostic feature. However, later studies have not supported this (Fleming and Johnson 1970; Perez et al. 1973) and current major studies are not utilizing weight as a staging feature (NWTS: unpublished results). Microscopic residual disease is presumed present when capsular invasion or invasion of perihilar tissue is noted by the pathologist. The significance of these features has been demonstrated (Knudson and Strong 1972; Kumar et al. 1975) and incorporated into most staging systems.

The importance of lymph node metastases (Breslow et al. 1978; Lemerle et al. 1976a; Perez et al. 1973) on overall prognosis has caused us to place this originally stage II feature into a stage III status. Regional lymph node metastasis was associated with a 10% 3-year survival by Perez (Perez et al. 1973). Breslow of the National Wilms' Tumor Study (NWTS) noted a three-fold increase in deaths with lymph node metastasis (Breslow et al. 1978). Lemerle et al. (1976a) noted a 50% reduction in survival when lymph nodes were obviously involved. Progress in treatment of Wilms' tumor recently has aimed at the reduction of radiation dosage and elimination of radiotherapy in certain stages of Wilms' tumor (NWTS: unpublished results). For this reason, features that have been particularly associated with abdominal recurrence have been placed in stage III so that radiotherapy would still be used (see Table 3.3). Lemerle noted a significant difference in survival between patients with or without tumor rupture and spillage, regional lymph node involvement, adhesions, and renal vein thrombosis and infiltration (Lemerle et al. 1976a). Perez et al. (1973) also noted similar poor prognostic features with regional lymph node involvement and renal vein invasion.

Beckwith's pathologic review of NWTS I has shown that sarcomatous or anaplastic histopathology had a 21% and 10% relapse-free 2-year survival respectively, a significantly poorer prognosis than the more common blastemal or epithelial types (Beckwith and Palmer 1978; Breslow et al. 1978). Studies by several pathologists have shown that survival decreases with the decrease in tubular epithelium and increase in sarcomatous and anaplastic features (Beckwith and Palmer 1978; Currie et al. 1973; Kheir et al. 1978; Lawler et al. 1975; Lemerle et al. 1976a). From Beckwith's review (Beckwith and Palmer 1978) the current NWTS III plans to treat all patients with unfavorable histology, (including renal sarcoma, diffuse and focal anaplasia) as stage IV disease regardless of prior staging criteria (NWTS: unpublished results). Beckwith divides the prognostic criteria according to which feature is predominant.

Pathology

Pathologic evaluation of renal tumors begins in the operating room as the surgeon hands the intact tumor to the pathologist. The surface of the intact kidney and tumor is examined for areas of tumor penetration through the capsule. The renal pelvis is inspected for invasion of peripelvic fact or renal vein. The tumor may be halved by a longitudinal cut through both poles and the pelvis. Sections are taken for special studies, electron microscopy, cytogenetic and immunologic or enzymatic assays. The tumor is then fixed in formalin for pathologic evaluation. Sections are taken from the vascular and ureteric margins and through the renal pelvis at the nearest and most distant points to the tumor. Multiple sections are taken at all areas suspicious of capsule penetration as well as randomly to evaluate the tumor histology and tumor capsule. Hilar lymph nodes are also sectioned to identify metastases. Biopsied lymph nodes or areas of suspected metastases are prepared and sectioned for study. The pathologist will confirm the stage from this accumulated material.

Recognition of multiple variants of Wilms' tumor has provided a basis for better understanding of the clinical features. Earlier reports of improved survival in children diagnosed during the first year of life (Harvey 1950; Klapproth 1959; Scott 1956) may be due to benign variants, such as mesoblastic nephroma and nephroblastomatosis, that occur predominantly in the first year of life (Sotelo-Avila and Gooch 1976). Table 3.4 lists the major variants encountered in pathologic evaluation of pediatric renal tumors.

Table 3.4. Pathologic variants of pediatric renal tumors

(1) Nodular renal blastema
(2) Nephroblastomatosis (diffuse)
(3) Mesoblastic nephroma
(4) Wilms' tumor — nephroblastoma
     (a) Typical (blastema, epithelial, mixed)
     (b) Cystic
     (c) Anaplastic (focal, diffuse)
     (d) Sarcomatous (rhabdomyosarcomatoid, clear cell, hyalinizing)

Nodular Renal Blastema and Diffuse Nephroblastomatosis

Nodular renal blastema, perhaps a primitive precursor of Wilms' tumor, has been noted as an incidental autopsy finding (Bove et al. 1969; Shanklin and Sotelo-Avila 1969) or on the opposite kidney when Wilms' tumor is diagnosed (Bove and McAdams 1978). It appears as a small pearly gray discrete nodule, sharply circumscribed but not encapsulated, just beneath the capsule of the kidney. Pathologic examination shows primitive undifferentiated cells with large hyperchromatic nuclei and scanty cytoplasm. These cells appear similar to the blastemal cell of Wilms' tumor (Bove et al. 1969). The areas may become confluent, encompassing the entire surface of both kidneys, and resulting in bilateral nephroblastomatosis. These lesions appear as massively enlarged kidneys with exaggerated fetal lobulations mimicking bilateral polycystic disease or bilateral Wilms' tumor (Chadarévian et al. 1977; Haddy et al. 1977; Kumar et al. 1978; Telander et al. 1978). Although clinically non-metastatic, these tumors are treated following biopsy with vincristine and dactinomycin, with or without radiotherapy, and usually the renal anatomy returns to normal (Chadarévian et al. 1977; Kumar et al. 1978; Telander et al. 1978). It is suspected that the lesions of nodular renal blastema may transform into Wilms' tumor because in patients with Wilms' tumor nodular renal blastema is found in separate areas of the involved kidney or in the opposite kidney (Bove et al. 1969; Bove and McAdams 1978; Kumar et al. 1978). Nodular renal blastema is associated with Wilms' tumor and is also more prominent in infants with trisomy 18 or with genitourinary anomalies, hemihypertrophy or Beckwith Wiedemann syndrome (Bove and McAdams 1978; Chadarevian et al. 1977; Haddy et al. 1977; Kumar et al. 1978).

Mesoblastic Nephroma

Mesoblastic nephroma, a benign renal tumor, is diagnosed most frequently in the first month of life. It has an excellent prognosis once nephrectomy has been performed (Bolande et al. 1967; Kay et al. 1966; Richmond and Dougall 1970). The tumor is an ovoid, yellow-gray rubbery mass that on cut section is whorled and trabeculated without hemorrhage or necrosis (Bolande et al. 1967). The tumor cells are elongated cigar-shaped spindles arranged in broad interlacing sheets. The tumor appears fibroblastic in origin with nests of abnormal tubules and glomeruli scattered within the tumor (Bolande et al. 1967). Metastasis has not been reported although local recurrence has been observed (Green and Jaffe 1978).

Deaths reported with mesoblastic nephroma have been attributed to the toxicity of chemotherapy and radiation; therefore, the only recommended treatment is complete surgical resection.

Wilms' Tumor

On gross examination, Wilms' tumor may arise at either pole or centrally within the kidney displacing and infiltrating normal renal structures. Separate satellite nodules may appear in the remaining kidney tissue. Bulging nodular masses may protrude from the tumor surface yet remain covered by the thick renal capsule. The tumor is generally white to gray white, fleshy and friable. Beneath the capsule and on cut section hemorrhage, cysts and areas of necrosis can be seen. Fibrous cords separate parts of the tumor, giving a lobular appearance.

The tumor may be of massive size yet still remain entirely encapsulated. Hemorrhage into the tumor or rapid cellular growth may double its size in a few days. The tumor may extend beyond the capsule, invading the adrenal, perinephric fat, diaphragm, liver or colon. It may invade the renal vein and into the vena cava with extension into the right atrium. Spread to perihilar and para-aortic lymph nodes is a common first site of metastasis.

Histologic examination demonstrates a variety of mesenchymal and epithelial cells in various stages of development. Renal blastemal cells, the major cell type, are primitive epithelial progenitors of the glomerulotubular cells. Spindle-shaped hyperchromatic cells appear in nodules surrounded by undifferentiated stroma. These cells may form structures resembling abortive glomeruli or as is more frequently seen, tubules of low cuboidal epithelial cells. In some areas these tubular epithelial cells may predominate. The embryonic mesenchymal origin of this tumor is suggested by the occasional presence of cartilaginous, adipose or striated muscle tissue.

Less typical histology may appear as areas of markedly anaplastic cells with bizarre nuclear features, or sheets of cells typical of sarcomas with polygonal form, abundant acidophilic cytoplasm, rounded nuclei and a central dark nucleolus. Less frequent cell types are the clear cell pattern, characterized by well-defined polygonal cells with water clear cytoplasm and rounded nuclei, and the hyalinizing pattern, characterized by a variably abundant intercellular matrix resembling malignant osteoid (Beckwith and Palmer 1978).

Histopathologic staging correlates well with survival. The importance of tubular differentiation has been noted by various authors (Breslow et al. 1978; Currie et al. 1973; Kheir et al. 1978; Lawler et al. 1975; Lemerle et al. 1976a; Perez et al. 1973). An abundance of well-differentiated tubular cells is associated with a better prognosis compared to undifferentiated sarcomatous or anaplastic features. The survival of patients by histologic type is presented in Table 3.5.

The problem in histopathologic staging is with the intermediate group of tumors, those showing fewer epithelial tubular structures (i.e. <50%) or areas of focal anaplasia and cellular atypia. Pathologists must agree on what histologic features should be seen in order to define this intermediate prognostic group. Focal anaplasia may be missed by one pathologist only to be seen in review by a second pathologist. The frequency of reporting focal anaplasia depends on the number of slides taken

Table 3.5.   Disease-free survival reports according to favorable and unfavorable histology.

	Favorable		Intermediate		Unfavorable	
	Patient surviving	% Surviving 2 years	Patient surviving	% Surviving 2 years	Patient surviving	% Surviving 2 years
Jereb and Sandstedt (1973)	12/16	75	16/65	25	6/31	19
Currie (1973)	5/5	100	4/6	66	1/10	10
Lawler (1975)	5/6	83	11/24	46	7/32	22[a]
Perez (1973)	6/10	60	6/9	67	7/24	23
Lemerle (1976)	20/22	90[b]	71/116	61[b]	20/46	43[b]
Kheir (1978)	7/7	100	7/9	77	3/10	30
Beckwith (1978)	338/364	93	9/15	60[c]	12/34	35
Total	393/430	91.3	124/244	50.8	56/193	29

[a] Combining two lower survival groups.
[b] 5-year survival instead of 2 year.
[c] Focal anaplasia group, said to be unfavorable by Beckwith.

and the individual pathologist's interpretation. The prognostic significance of the unfavorable histologies, diffuse anaplasia and sarcomatous variant, has been shown, but the importance of focal anaplasia remains to be elucidated. Beckwith and Palmer (1978) reported that unfavorable histology (including the intermediate group with focal anaplasia) accounted for 11% of all Wilms' tumor. Thus only one to three such cases are diagnosed at any one institution per year.

It is speculated that the sarcomatous variant which is similar to rhabdomyosarcoma and can metastasize to unusual sites, the brain and bones, may be a separate tumor entity (Marsden and Lawler 1978; Penchansky and Gallo 1979). However, closer inspection of these tumors reveals that blastemal and epithelial elements may be scattered in foci throughout the primary tumor and metastases may have either sarcomatous, blastemal or epithelial components.

Treatment

The current therapy for Wilms' tumor is the result of a cooperative effort of surgeons, radiotherapists and clinical oncologists who have created coordinated treatment plans which provide evaluable information on clinical effectiveness of each phase of therapy. Further questions are being asked by treatment programs to find the optimal survival with a minimal treatment morbidity. Whenever an exploration of the abdomen is anticipated in a child with an abdominal mass, the surgeon should be cognizant of the surgical procedure as well as the overall treatment plan.

Successful treatment of Wilms' tumor began with advances in surgical techniques. Between 1900 and 1960, surgical management of Wilms' tumor altered the prognosis from a uniformly fatal disease to 40% 2-year survival (Gross and Neuhauser 1950). Advances in pediatric anesthesiology, postoperative care and antibiotics contributed to the improved survival. Abeshouse (1957) determined from his survey of physicians that the cure rate for surgery varied from 5% to 44%. One of the highest cure rates was reported by Gross and Neuhauser (1950) from Boston. A major feature of the Boston program was the emphasis on removing the tumor without rupture or biopsy and the use of the transabdominal approach (Farber 1966).

From 1920 to 1960, radiotherapy was evaluated for preoperative reduction of tumor bulk or postoperative treatment of residual tumor (Abeshouse 1957; Harvey 1950; Klapproth 1959; Scott 1956). Control of local disease became possible, but deaths due to pulmonary metastasis remained the major problem. In 1950, Harvey reviewed the cumulative data of 44 publications demonstrating that with surgery alone or radiotherapy alone survival rates were only 15%, but a combination of these two treatments gave a 30% survival. In contrast, Klapproth (1959) reviewed 135 cases from the literature of 1940–1958 and noted that the 20% survival with surgery alone was similar to the 27% survival with surgery plus irradiation. In addition, Gross and Ladd believed that preoperative radiotherapy was not essential, that it delayed surgical removal, and perhaps allowed time for tumor metastasis (Farber 1966). Preoperative radiotherapy or chemotherapy risks misdiagnosis and does not improve disease-free survival (Chadarévian et al. 1977; Green and Jaffe 1978; Kay ct al. 1966). Once its value was determined, radiotherapy dosages up to 5000 rads were given as the only therapy or in conjunction with surgery. Local control of tumor was achieved but frequently at a cost of deformities of the spine, and liver and kidney damage (Arneil et al. 1974; Mitus et al. 1969; Probert and Parker 1975; Tefft et al. 1970). With the use of chemotherapy, particularly dactinomycin, dosages were reduced to 2400–3000 rads (Farber 1966).

The development of successful chemotherapy began with treatment of metastatic disease. Farber et al. (1960) demonstrated clinical response of metastatic tumors to dactinomycin with a 37% survival in a population of patients that previously would have died. A trial of dactinomycin and radiation in patients without extra-abdominal metastases at diagnosis resulted in an 87% survival (Farber et al. 1960). Fernbach and Martyn (1966) confirmed these early studies by obtaining a 92% survival with surgery, postoperative irradiation and dactinomycin.

Vincristine sulfate was also being evaluated in the early 1960s. In 1963, Sutow et al. reported temporary response of metastatic Wilms' tumor to vincristine in 8 of 12 children. A combination of pulmonary and abdominal irradiation with vincristine employed by Vietti et al. (1970) resulted in a complete regression of metastatic disease in 73% of their patients and a 45% 2-year survival.

The National Wilms' Tumor Study I demonstrated the effectiveness of the combination of these two agents. In stage II and III patients, dactinomycin alone resulted in a 67% 2-year survival compared to 72% for vincristine. However, administration of both of the agents resulted in an 82% 2-year survival (D'Angio et al. 1976), surpassing all single drug studies (Green and Neuhauser 1950; Lemerle et al. 1976a). At St. Jude Hospital, 26 patients seen from 1968–1972 with all stages of Wilms' tumor were treated with this combination and 16 survived.

From Neuhauser's previous work on the effects of radiation (Neuhauser et al. 1952), D'Angio (1968) devised a sliding scale for radiation doses adjusted for age. This provided infants less than 18 months old with less than the 'optimal' 2400 rads (D'Angio 1968; D'Angio et al. 1978; Neuhauser et al. 1952). Hussey demonstrated that, when combined with chemotherapy, doses of radiation below 2400 rads resulted in the same control of tumor recurrence as higher doses (Hussey et al. 1971). Aron (1974) confirmed this observation with doses as low as 1500–1800 rads (600–725 ret). Our group and the NWTS are evaluating lower doses of irradiation or no irradiation for some cases. This is because intra-abdominal recurrence accounted for only 22% of all relapses and involved only 6.7% of all patients treated for Groups IA, II and III in NWTS I (D'Angio et al. 1978). The dose of irradiation did not appear to influence the frequency of abdominal recurrence (NWTS: unpublished results). NWTS II demonstrated that for stage I Wilms' tumor, the combination of vincristine and dactinomycin was as effective as radiation in preventing abdominal recurrence

Table 3.6. Treatment schema of the Second National Wilms' Tumor Study. Although more advanced protocols are now in use, this design well illustrates the type of multimodal therapy employed. Such treatment should only be conducted at specialized centers since its potential toxicity is severe.

Postoperative regimen by stage of disease
Stage I — no radiotherapy. Dactinomycin and vincristine[a].
Stages II–IV — radiotherapy plus dactinomycin and vincristine[a].

Follow-up chemotherapy
Randomization to one of four arms:
(E) Dact + VCR[b] at 6 weeks and 3, 6 months.
(F) Dact + VCR at 6 weeks and 3, 6, 9, 12, 15 months.
(C) VCR at 6, 7, 8 weeks.
     Dact + VCR at 3, 6, 9, 12, 15 months
(D) VCR at 6, 7, 8 weeks.
     Dact + VCR at 3, 6, 9, 12, 15 months.
     ADR at 6 weeks and 4.5, 7.5, 10.5, 13.5 months[c].

Dact = dactinomycin; actinomycin D.
 VCR = vincristine.
ADR = adriamycin; doxorubicin.
[a] Dact 15 mcg/kg/day × 5 (maximum 500 mcg/day).
 VCR 1.5 mg/m²/day, days 7, 14, 21, 28, 35 (maximum 2.0 mg dose).
[b] Dact 15 mcg/kg/day × 5 (maximum 500 mcg/day).
 VCR 1.5 mg/m²/day, days 1 and 5.
[c] ADR 60 mg/m² × 1 day.

and there is over 90% disease-free survival (NWTS: unpublished results). Details of this trial are outlined in Table 3.6. This trial, and more advanced studies which have replaced it, well exemplify the multiple modalities and multiple-drug regimens necessary to improve results in Wilms' tumor. It should be emphasized that such treatment programs are potentially hazardous and are best administered at specialized centers. The necessity for irradiation to eradicate microscopic residual disease currently is being evaluated in several studies.

The next major advance in chemotherapy has been the use of doxorubicin (adriamycin). Impressive in early reports for a variety of malignancies (Bellani et al. 1975; Bonadonna et al. 1970; Tan et al. 1973), adriamycin was studied by six oncology groups for Wilms' tumor. Cumulative data, reported by Tan et al. (1975), showed a 67% (31 out of 46) incidence of complete or partial response to adriamycin. In NWTS II the addition of adriamycin for stage II–IV Wilms' tumor resulted in improved survival for stage II–III patients with unfavorable histology and for all stage IV patients (NWTS: unpublished results). From 1972 to 1979, the authors treated 61 patients with vincristine, dactinomycin, adriamycin and irradiation for stage II–IV disease. Forty-four have been followed for >2 years and 36 survive (82%). Of the eight deaths, three were associated with non-tumor complications (*Pneumocystis carinii* pneumonia, volvulus, accident) and a fourth patient died of renal failure due to bilateral renal involvement (Table 3.7).

The clinical response of Wilms' tumor to chemotherapeutic agents other than vincristine, dactinomycin and adriamycin has been disappointing. Cyclophosphamide, which appears to have little activity against Wilms' tumor (Sutow 1967), has been added to the NWTS III therapy for stage IV Wilms' tumor and all tumors with unfavorable histology (NWTS: unpublished results), because of recent success with a combination of cyclophosphamide, vinblastine and high-dose dactinomycin (Ortega et al. 1979). Other chemotherapeutic agents are being studied but the generally favorable prognosis in Wilms' tumor limits large scale trials of new agents.

Table 3.7. SJCRH — Study II — Wilms' tumor, 1973–1979, 61 patients

Stage	Alive >2 years	Alive <2 years	Dead	Total
I	4	6	2[a]	12
II	10	6	0	16
III	14	2	3[b]	19
IV	3	1	3[c]	7
V	5[d]	1[d]	1[e]	7
	36	16	9	61

[a] One patient died with anaplastic variant.
  One patient died NED-volvulus.
[b] One patient Px — in 1978 and died with anaplastic variant.
  One patient died of sudden unknown cause 2 years off therapy.
  One patient died of liver metastasis and liver failure.
[c] One patient died of *Pneumocystis carinii* pneumonitis 5 months into therapy.
  Two patients died of recurrence of pulmonary metastasis.
[d] Four of seven patients with bilateral disease had accompanying nephroblastomatosis.
[e] Died in renal failure.
SJCRH — St. Jude Children's Research Hospital Memphis Tennessee.

Bilateral Wilms' Tumor

Despite the sensitivity of Wilms' tumor to therapy, a serious problem exists when the tumor presents in both kidneys. The frequency of bilateral Wilms' tumor averages 4.7% (Table 3.3) but ranges from 0 to 11% in reported series (Bishop et al. 1977; Bond 1975; Jereb and Sandstedt 1973; Knudson and Strong 1972; Lemerle et al. 1976a; Ragab et al. 1972). The median age at diagnosis is <2 years, slightly younger than for unilateral Wilms' tumor (Knudson and Strong 1972). The diagnosis of bilateral Wilms' tumor may be immediately apparent with initial physical examination and radiographic studies or not until the surgeon examines the contralateral kidney. Palpation and inspection of the opposite 'uninvolved' kidney may disclose unsuspected tumor nodules. Subsequent development of tumor in the remaining kidney can be detected by intravenous urography and ultrasound performed periodically during therapy. About 35% of bilateral cases occur as later involvement of the contralateral kidney from a few months to 10 years after diagnosis (Ragab et al. 1972).

The child who presents with massive bilateral tumors presents special problems requiring a thorough clinical and radiographic evaluation followed by an individualized treatment program. Intravenous urography, ultrasonography, and renal arteriography can frequently define the size and location of the tumor and the remaining functional kidney. With this information, an operation can be designed to provide maximum preservation of renal function. Several approaches have given similar results, including nephrectomy of the more involved kidney plus heminephrectomy or biopsy, bilateral heminephrectomy or bilateral biopsy with second look surgery. The combination of chemotherapy and low dosage (1200–1500 rads) radiation has resulted in 2-year disease-free survivals of 87% in NWTS I (Bishop et al. 1977) and 80% in our series demonstrating that this is a far from hopeless condition.

Prognosis

In 1980, the child with Wilms' tumor entering a coordinated treatment program has an 80%–90% chance of cure. Data from the study by the Medical Research Council in the U.K. (1970–1973) demonstrated that patients in organized clinical studies have a 3-year survival of 77% compared to 58% for patients treated randomly (Lennox et al. 1979). Disease-free survival for 2–3 years generally indicates eradication of the tumor, since <5% of patients relapse after 2 years (Breslow et al. 1978; Platt and Linden 1964).

Important prognostic factors for patients with Wilms' tumor have evolved as clinical trials progressively improved survival. Age of the patient was initially felt to be a significant factor in both European (Ledlie et al. 1970; Lemerle et al. 1976a) and the NWTS I studies (Breslow et al. 1978), with children younger than 2 years old more likely to survive. An explanation was Aron's (1974) finding that tumors were more often nonmetastatic in patients younger than 2 years old. Later studies in Britain (Bond 1975; Lennox et al. 1979; Marsden and Steward 1968; Morris Jones et al. 1978; Richmond and Dougall 1970) and the United States (Fleming and Johnson 1970; Perez et al. 1973) have shown no relationship between age and survival. Fleming and Johnson (1970) found that the stage of disease predicted survival better than age.

The staging system based on pathologic features also predicts survival. Factors influencing survival include capsular or perihilar invasion, lymph node involvement, peritoneal seeding and distant metastases. Other features such as weight or volume of tumor (Breslow et al. 1978; Garcia et al. 1963) have not been confirmed as significant prognostic factors (NWTS: unpublished results).

The influence of histology on prognosis was conclusively demonstrated by a review of the pathology of Wilms' tumor in NWTS I (Beckwith and Palmer 1978). Sarcomatous and anaplastic variants constituted 11.5% of all Wilms' tumors studied but accounted for 51.9% of all deaths. The patients' 2-year survival with sarcomatous and diffuse anaplastic variants were 36% and 20% respectively. Therefore, patients with these variants of Wilms' tumor have a poor prognosis regardless of stage or other prognostic factors. However, the significance of focal anaplasia is unclear and requires further study.

Metastatic disease at diagnosis, once considered uniformly fatal, is responsive to surgery, radiation and chemotherapy and nearly 50% of these patients attain 2-year disease-free survival (NWTS: unpublished results). Although pulmonary metastases account for 81% of all relapses (Breslow et al. 1978), these lesions and abdominal metastases may remain amenable to surgical resection (Wedemeyer et al. 1968), irradiation (Cassady et al. 1977; Monson et al. 1972) and/or combination chemotherapy (Ortega et al. 1979). The availability of new surgical techniques, diagnostic imaging procedures and newer chemotherapeutic agents in major cancer centers promises further improvement in survival for these patients.

Summary

Therapy of Wilms' tumor has advanced steadily from a 20%–40% survival with surgery alone to 80% survival today with a combined approach. Transabdominal surgery followed by the judicious use of radiotherapy and multiagent chemotherapy provides the basis for modern therapy. The surgeon, pathologist and diagnostic radiologist provide essential information for staging and appropriate therapy. This cooperation provides an excellent probability of survival for their patients. Current therapeutic studies are attempting to safely reduce therapy for those patients with a favorable prognosis and intensify therapeutic efforts for the patient with an unfavorable prognosis.

References

Abeshouse BS (1957) Management of Wilms' tumor by national survey and review of the literature. J Urol 77: 792–813

Arneil GC, Emanual IG, Flatman GE (1974) Nephritis in two children after irradiation and chemotherapy for nephroblastoma. Lancet I: 960–963

Aron BS (1974) Wilms' tumor — A clinical study of eighty-one patients. Cancer 33: 637–646

Baert L, Verduyn H, Vereecken R (1966) Wilms' tumor (nephroblastoma): Report of 57 histologically proved cases. J Urol 96: 871–874

Barakat AY, Papadopoulou ZL, Chandra RS, Hollerman CE, Calcagno PL (1974) Pseudohermaphroditism, nephron disorder and Wilms' tumor: A unifying concept. Pediatrics 54: 366–369

Beckwith JB, Palmer NF (1978) Histopathology and prognosis of Wilms' tumor. Cancer 41: 1937–1948

Betkerur U, Lanzkowsky P (1977) Pleural effusion in Wilms' tumor. J Pediatr Surg 12: 523–525

Bellani FF, Gasparini M, Bonadonna G (1975) Adriamycin in Wilms' tumor previously treated with chemotherapy. Eur J Cancer 11: 593–595

Bishop HC, Tefft M, Evans AE, D'Angio GJ (1977) Survival in bilateral Wilms' tumor — Review of 30 national Wilms' tumor study cases. J Pediatr Surg 12: 631–638

Bolande RP, Brough AJ, Izant RJ Jr (1967) Congenital mesoblastic nephroma of infancy. Pediatrics 40: 272–278

Bonadonna G, Monfardini S, DeLana M, Fossati-Bellini F, Beretta G (1970) Phase I and preliminary phase II evaluation of adriamycin. Cancer Res 30: 2572–2582

Bond JV (1975) Prognosis and treatment of Wilms' tumor at Great Ormond Street Hospital for Sick Children 1960–1972. Cancer 36: 1202–1207

Bove KE, McAdams AJ (1978) Multifocal nephroblastic neoplasia. J Natl Cancer Inst 61: 285–289

Bove KE, Koffler H, McAdams AJ (1969) Nodular renal blastema. Cancer 24: 232–332

Bradley JE, Pincoffs MC (1938) The association of adeno-myo-sarcoma of the kidney (Wilms' tumor) with arterial hypertension. Ann Intern Med 11: 1613–1628

Breslow NE, Palmer NF, Hill LR, Buring Jr, D'Angio GJ (1978) Wilms' tumor: Prognostic factors for patients without metastases at diagnosis. Cancer 41: 1577–1589

Cassady JR, Tefft M, Filler RM, Jaffe N, Hellman S (1973) Considerations in the radiation therapy of Wilms' tumor. Cancer 32: 598–608

Cassady JR, Jaffe N, Filler RM (1977) The increasing importance of radiation therapy in the improved prognosis of children with Wilms' tumor. Cancer 39: 825–829

Chadarevian JP, Fletcher BD, Chattes Jr, Rabinovitch HH (1977) Massive infantile nephroblastomatosis. Cancer 39: 2294–2305

Cochran W, Froggart P (1967) Bilateral nephroblastoma in two sisters. J Urol 97: 216–220

Currie DP, Daly JT, Grimes JH, Anderson EE (1973) Wilms' tumor: A clinical pathological correlation. J Urol 109: 495–500

D'Angio GJ (1968) Radiation therapy in Wilms' tumor. JAMA 204: 987–988

D'Angio GJ, Evans AE, Breslow N (1976) The treatment of Wilms' tumor — Results of the national Wilms' tumor study. Cancer 38: 633–646

D'Angio GJ, Tefft M, Breslow N, Meyer JA (1978) Radiation therapy of Wilms' tumor: Results according to dose, field, post-operative timing and histology. Int J Rad Oncology Biol Phys 4: 769–780

Everson RB, Fraumeni JR Jr (1975) Declining mortality and improving survival from Wilms' tumor. Med Ped Oncology 1: 3–10

Farber S (1966) Chemotherapy in the treatment of leukemia and Wilms' tumor. JAMA 198: 826–836

Farber S, D'Angio G, Evans A, Mitus A (1969) Clinical studies of actinomycin D with special reference to Wilms' tumor in children. Ann NY Acad Sci 89: 421–425

Fernbach DJ, Martyn DT (1966) Role of dactinomycin in the improved survival of children with Wilms' tumor. JAMA 195: 1005–1009

Fleming ID, Johnson WW (1970) Clinical and pathologic staging as a guide in the management of Wilms' tumor. Cancer 26: 660–665

Fraumeni JF Jr, Glass AG (1968) Wilms' tumor and congenital aniridia. JAMA 206: 825–828

Fraumeni JF Jr, Geiser CF, Manning MD (1967) Wilms' tumor and congenital hemihypertrophy: Report of five new cases and review of literature. Pediatrics 40: 886–899

Ganguly A, Gribble J, Tune B, Kempson RL, Luetscher JA (1973) Renin-secreting Wilms' tumor with severe hypertension. Ann Int Med 79: 835–837

Garcia M, Douglass C, Schlosser JV (1963) Classification and prognosis in Wilms' tumor. Radiology 80: 574–580

Green DM, Jaffe N (1978) Wilms' tumor — Model of a curable pediatric malignant solid tumor. Cancer Treat Rev 5: 143–172

Green DM, Jaffe N (1979) The role of chemotherapy in the treatment of Wilms' tumor. Cancer 44: 52–57

Gross RE, Neuhauser EBD (1950) Treatment of mixed tumors of the kidney in childhood. Pediatrics 6: 843–852

Haddy TB, Bailie MD, Bernstein J, Kaufman DB, Rous SN (1977) Bilateral diffuse nephroblastomatosis: Report of a case managed with chemotherapy. J Pediatr 90: 784–786

Harvey RM (1950) Wilms' tumor: Evaluation of treatment methods. Radiology 54: 689–699

Hussey DH, Castro JR, Sullivan MP, Sutow WW (1971) Radiation therapy in management of Wilms' tumor. Radiology 101: 663–668

Jaffe N, Jockin H, Tefft M, Traggis D, Filler RM (1973) Wilms' tumor: Diagnosis by thoracentesis. Chest 64: 130–132

Jereb B, Sandstedt B (1973) Structure and size versus prognosis in nephroblastoma. Cancer 31: 1473–1481

Kay S, Pratt CB, Salzberg AM (1966) Hamartoma (leiomyomatous type) of the kidney. Cancer 19: 1825–1832

Kheir S, Pritchett PS, Moreno H, Robinson CA (1978) Histologic grading of Wilms' tumor as a potential prognostic factor: Results of a retrospective study of 26 patients. Cancer 41: 1199–1207

Klapproth HJ (1959) Wilms' tumor: A report of 45 cases and an analysis of 1351 cases reported in world's literature from 1940–1958. J Urol 81: 633–648

Knudson AG, Strong LC (1972) Mutation and cancer: A model for Wilms' tumor of the kidney. J Natl Cancer Inst 48: 313–324

Kumar APM, Hutsu O, Fleming ID, et al. (1975) Capsular and vascular invasion: Important prognostic factors in Wilms' tumor. J Pediatr Surg 10: 301–309

Kumar APM, Pratt CB, Coburn TP, Johnson WW (1978) Treatment strategy for nodular renal blastema and nephroblastomatosis associated with Wilms' tumor. J Pediatr Surg 13: 281–285

Lawler W, Marsden HB, Palmer MK (1975) Wilms' tumor histologic variation and prognosis. Cancer 36: 1122–1126

Ledlie EM, Mynors LS, Draper GJ, Gorbach PD (1970) Natural history and treatment of Wilms' tumour: An analysis of 335 cases occurring in England and Wales 1962–6. Br Med J iv: 195–200

Lermerle J, Tournade MF, Ferard-Marchant R (1976a) Wilms' tumor: Natural history and prognostic factors. Cancer 37: 2667–2566

Lemerle J, Voute PA, Tournade MF (1976b) Preoperative versus postoperative radiotherapy, single versus multiple courses of actinomycin D, in the treatment of Wilms' tumor. Cancer 38: 647–654

Lennox EL, Stiller CA, Morris-Jones PH, Wilson LMK (1979) Nephroblastoma: Treatment during 1970–3 and the effect on survival of inclusion in the first MRC trial. Br Med J ii: 567–569

Lines DR (1968) Nephrotic syndrome and nephroblastoma. J Pediatr 72: 264–265

Marsden HB, Steward JK (1968) Problems of children's tumours in Britain. Recent Results Cancer Res 10: 1–13

Marsden HB, Steward JK (1968) Renal tumours. Recent Results Cancer Res 10: 327–361

Marsden HB, Lawler W (1978) Bone-metastasizing renal tumour of childhood. Br J Cancer 38: 437–441

Miller RW, Fraumeni JF Jr, Manning MD (1964) Association of Wilms' tumor with aniridia, hemihypertrophy, and other congenital malformations. N Engl J Med 270: 922–927

Mitus A, Tefft M, Fellers FX (1969) Long term follow-up of renal functions of 108 children who underwent nephrectomy for malignant disease. Pediatrics 44: 912–921

Monson KJ, Brand WN, Boggs JD (1972) Results of small field irradiation of apparent solitary metastasis from Wilms' tumor. Radiology 104: 157–160

Morris Jones PH, Pearson D, Johnson AL (1978) Management of nephroblastoma in childhood. Arch Dis Child 53: 112–119

Neuhauser EBD, Willenborg MH, Berman CZ, Cohen J (1952) Irradiation effects of roentgen therapy on the growing spine. Radiology 59: 637–650

Ortega JA, Higgins GR, Williams K, Siegel SE, Hays DM (1979) Vincristine, actinomycin D, and cytoxan (VAC) chemotherapy for recurrent metastatic Wilms' tumor in previously treated children. (Abstract) Proc AACR/ASCO 20: 341

Penchansky L, Gallo G (1979) Rhabdomyosarcoma of the kidney in children. Cancer 44: 285–292

Pendergrass TW (1976) Congenital anomalies in children with Wilms' tumor. Cancer 37: 403–409

Perez CA, Kaiman HA, Keith J (1973) Treatment of Wilms' tumor and factors affecting prognosis. Cancer 32: 609–617

Perlman M, Levin M, Wittels B (1975) Syndrome of fetal gigantism, renal hamartomas, and nephroblastomatosis with Wilms' tumor. Cancer 35: 1212–1217

Platt BB, Linden G (1964) Wilms' tumor — A comparison of 2 criteria for survival. Cancer 17: 1573–1578

Probert JC, Parker BR (1975) The effects of radiation therapy on bone growth. Radiology 114: 155–162

Ragab AH, Vietti TJ, Crist W, Perez C, McAllister W (1972) Bilateral Wilms' tumor. Cancer 30: 983–988

Ricardi VM, Sujansky E, Smith AC, Francke U (1978) Chromosomal imbalance in the aniridia-Wilms' tumor association: 11p interstitial deletion. Pediatrics 61: 604–608

Richmond H, Dougall AJ (1970) Neonatal renal tumors. J Pediatr Surg 5: 413–417

Rous SM, Bailie MD, Kaufman DB, Haddy TB, Mattson JC (1976) Nodular renal blastoma, nephroblastomatosis and Wilms' tumor: Different points on the same disease spectrum? Urology 8: 599–604

Sanyal SK, Saldivar V, Coburn TP, Wrenn EL, Kumar M (1976) Hyperdynamic heart failure due to A–V fistula associated with Wilms' tumor. Pediatrics 57: 564–568

Schullinger JN, Santulli TV, Casarella WJ, MacMillan RW (1977) Wilms' tumor: The role of right heart angiography in the management of selected cases. Ann Surg 185: 451–455

Scott LS (1956) Wilms' tumour: Its treatment and prognosis. Br Med J i: 200–203

Shanklin DR, Sotelo-Avila C (1969) In situ tumors in fetuses, newborns and young infants. Biol Neonate 14: 286–316

Slovis TL, Cushing B, Reilly BJ (1978) Wilms' tumor to the heart: Clinical and radiographic evaluation. AJR 131: 263–266

Sotelo-Avila C, Gooch WM (1976) Neoplasms associated with Beckwith–Wiedemann syndrome. Perspect Pediatr Pathol 3: 255–272

Spear GS, Hyde TP, Gruppo RA, Slosser R (1971) Pseudohermaphroditism, glomerulonephritis with the nephrotic syndrome and Wilms' tumor in infancy. J Pediatr 79: 677–681

Sukarochana K, Tolentino W, Kresewetter WB (1972) Wilms' tumor and hypertension. J Pediatr Surg 7: 573–578

Sutow WW, (1965) Chemotherapy in childhood cancer (except leukemia) An appraisal. Cancer 18: 1585–89

Sutow WW (1967) Cyclophosphamide (NSC-26271) in Wilms tumor and rhabdomyosarcoma. Cancer Chemother Rep 51: 407–409

Sutow WW, Thurman WG, Windmiller J (1963) Vincristine (leurocristine) sulfate in the treatment of children with metastatic Wilms' tumor. Pediatrics 32: 880–887

Sutow WW, Hussey DH, Ayala AG, Sullivan MO (1977) Wilms' tumor. In: Sutow WW, Vietti TJ, Fernbach DJ (eds) Clinical pediatric oncology. Mosby, St Louis, pp 538–568

Tan C, Etcubanas E, Wollner N (1973) Adriamycin — An antitumor antibiotic in the treatment of neoplastic diseases. Cancer 32: 9–17

Tan C, Rosen G, Ghavimi F (1975) Adriamycin (NSC-123127) in pediatric malignancies. Cancer Chemother Rep [3] 6: 259–266

Tefft M, Mitus A, Dos L, Vawter GF, Filler RM (1970) Irradiation of the liver in children: Review of experience in the acute and chronic phases, and in the intact normal and partially resected. AJR 108: 365–385

Telander RL, Gilchrist GS, Burgert O, Kelalis PP, Goellner JR (1978) Bilateral massive nephroblastomatosis in infancy. J Pediatr Surg 13: 163–168

Vietti TJ, Sullivan MP, Haggard ME, Holcomb TM, Berry DH (1970) Vincristine sulfate and radiation therapy in metastatic Wilms' tumor. Cancer 25: 12–20

Wedemeyer PP, White JG, Nesbit ME (1968) Resection of metastases in Wilms' tumor: A report of three cases cured of pulmonary and hepatic metastases. Pediatrics 41: 446–451

Wilms M (1899) Die Mischgechwulste der Niere. Arthur Georgi, Leipzig, pp 1–90

Young JL, Miller RW (1975) Incidence of malignant tumors in U.S. children. J Pediatr 86: 254–258

Chapter 4

Primary Carcinoma of the Renal Pelvis and Ureter

B. S. Kasimis

Introduction

Tumors of the renal pelvis are relatively rare in comparison to neoplasms that arise from the renal parenchyma. In general, they comprise 7%–8% of all malignant renal tumors (Bloom et al. 1970; Lucke and Schlumberger 1957). However, significant variation of geographic distribution has been noted. In Yugoslavia particularly, where an extremely high frequency was found, an association with endemic nephropathy appears to be well established (Petkovic 1975). Some environmental factors associated with bladder cancer, i.e., cigarette smoking, probably coffee drinking, and work with leather, are also related to cancer of the renal pelvis and ureter (Armstrong et al. 1976; Schmauz and Cole 1974). Prolonged abuse of phenacetin has been linked to the development of pelvic and ureteric tumors affecting predominantly the female population of certain countries (Armstrong et al. 1976; Johansson and Wahlquist 1977). The average age of the patients varies between 60 and 70 years and the ratio of incidence in males versus females is approximately 2:1. A rare familial form of multiple transitional cell carcinomas has been described recently (Gittes 1978).

Pathology

The urinary tract is covered throughout by transitional epithelium or 'urothelium', and has common embryologic and functional features. Therefore, tumors of the renal pelvis, ureter and bladder share common clinical features that are dissimilar to those of renal parenchymal tumors (Resseguie et al. 1978). In men, the occurrence of associated bladder and ureteric tumors is more common than that of pelvic tumors alone, while in women the opposite is true. In patients with a primary tumor of the pelvis and ureter a history of previous bladder malignancy is present in approximately 40% (Batata and Grabstald 1976; Resseguie et al. 1978). In a series of 27 patients the ureteric tumors were more common on the left side where 63% were found and the lower third of the ureter was the site involved in 70% of the cases (Ghazi et al. 1979). Approximately 2% of tumors of the renal pelvis and ureter were found to be bilateral (Mazeman 1976). Synchronous or asynchronous development of multiple urothelial cancer is not uncommon.

In several large series (Johansson et al. 1976; Mazeman 1976; Wagle et al. 1974), the majority of the patients develop typical transitional cell carcinoma (90%) while a small number of other histological types, i.e., epidermoid carcinoma (8%), adeno-carcinoma, carcinosarcoma, melanoma, sarcoma, etc. has also been described. However, a possible fundamental difference exists in the pathogenesis of squamous cell carcinoma and adenocarcinoma where a highly significant association between these tumors and stone disease with or without infection has been documented. The above varieties are considered to arise secondarily to chronic irritation and subsequent metaplasia of the urothelium (Donnelly and Koontz 1975; Quattlebaum 1968).

Rarely, true benign polyps covered by normal urothelium exist, with histo-pathological features distinct from papillary tumors.

Leukoplakia of the urothelium is uncommon but rare reports stress the import-ance of this lesion that is generally considered to be premalignant and a step further down the line of squamous metaplasia (Reece and Koontz 1975). A few cases of carcinoma in situ have been reported but the scanty data preclude any definitive statement about the natural history or treatment of these lesions (Khan et al. 1979).

The lymphatic drainage of the renal pelvis and ureter is diffuse and not well defined, and early involvement by tumors of small size but high histologic grade is not unusual. Spread is usually to adjacent organs, i.e., kidneys, adrenal glands, pancreas, spleen, lumbar and sacral vertebrae. Nonetheless more distant meta-stases are usually found in the lungs, liver and bones.

Clinical Presentation and Diagnosis

Hematuria is the most common presenting symptom, occurring in 60%–95% of cases. The bleeding is usually gross and painless. The next most common symptoms are flank pain (24%), urinary frequency (10%), fever, weight loss, palpable mass, or other symptoms usually associated with concomitant bladder cancer (Batata and Grabstald 1976). Although there is no distinct difference in the overall clinical picture between renal pelvis and ureteric carcinoma, urinary tract infections are more common in the former type (Resseguie et al. 1978). The average time from the onset of symptoms until diagnosis has been 5–12 months. However, the frequent concomitant presence of bladder tumors with either pelvic or ureteric carcinoma creates certain diagnostic difficulties. The classic triad of gross hematuria, palpable mass and non- or poorly-functioning kidney on excretory urogram, supposed to be pathognomonic for the disease, is extraordinarily rare (Ochsner et al. 1974). More commonly found (19.2%) is the triad of hematuria, pain and abdominal mass (Wagle et al. 1974).

In general, pelvic and ureteric tumors are diagnosed by intravenous urograms (IVU). In order of frequency, the most common findings for renal pelvic tumors are filling defect, hydronephrosis and non-visualization of the affected kidney. However, 2.5% of patients present with a normal IVU, while some pelvic neoplasms are indis-tinguishable from parenchymal tumors. For these rare cases, in addition to retrograde uretero-pyelography, arteriography can aid in establishing the correct pre-operative diagnosis (Pollen et al. 1975). Non-functioning kidneys have been found in association with low grade papillary tumors as well as with extensive infiltrating carcinomas, and lack of kidney visualization on IVU does not correlate with the tumor stage (Wagle et al. 1974). With ureteric tumors however, the order of frequency for the IVU findings is different. Batata et al. (1975) reported that nonvisualization was present in 46%, hydronephrosis with or without hydroureter in

34% and a ureteric filling defect with or without hydronephrosis or hydroureter in 19%. Retrograde uretero-pyelography has significantly aided in the diagnosis of ureteric tumors particularly those that are associated with minimal or no dilatation of the ureter, as well as those tumors located in the lower third of the ureter which are most difficult to diagnose. Angiography also can provide additional data in cases of inadequate visualization (Boijsen 1962). The diagnostic role of abdominal computerized tomography is currently being studied in several centers.

The contribution of urine cytology to screening and diagnosis of urothelial tumors remains at best controversial. The overall positivity remains low (29%–58%) while false negative results are not rare (Wagle et al. 1974; Donnelly and Koontz 1975; Batata et al. 1975; Eriksson and Johansson 1976). It is notable that positive cytology usually indicates the presence of higher tumor grades (Eriksson and Johansson 1976).

Brush biopsy introduced by Gill in 1973, appears to be useful in selected cases where cytology has been negative or indicative of low grade malignancy as well as in the preoperative differential diagnosis of certain benign abnormalities (Gittes 1978). In the rare instances of a pedunculated narrow stalk filling defect of the ureter that is associated with negative cytology and brush biopsy the suspicion of a benign polypoid lesion should be raised.

In rare cases of paraneoplastic hypercalcemia, the parathormone level was elevated markedly (Mandell et al. 1977).

Staging

Several staging systems have been proposed by various investigators, however, Grabstald et al. in 1971 introduced the most commonly used system that takes into account stage as well as histologic grade and divides the pelvic tumors into the following four groups:

Group 1 Histologically benign papilloma.
Group 2 Low stage carcinomas. These are usually of low grade and either without demonstrable invasion or with questionable or microfocal invasion or papillomas with carcinoma in situ either within the papilloma or elsewhere in the renal pelvic mucosa.
Group 3 High stage carcinomas; usually of high grade and infiltrating the renal pelvis or parenchyma but not extending beyond the kidney proper.
Group 4 High stage cancers invading outside the kidney parenchyma, including peripelvic and perirenal fat, lymph nodes, hilar blood vessels or adjacent or distant organs.

The four groups were subdivided as follows:

A Those without other tumors in the bladder or ureter.
B Those with other tumors in the bladder or ureter.

Tumor stage has been uniformly accepted as the most significant single prognostic factor and generally superior to grade. Frequently, excellent correlation between stage and grade has been found (Grabstald et al. 1971; Johansson et al. 1976).

Batata et al. 1975, following Jewett's staging system in bladder cancer, proposed a similar staging system for carcinoma of the ureter based on macroscopic and micro-scopic extent of invasion into the ureteric wall: stage A, submucosal infiltration; stage B, muscular invasion; stage C, periureteric fat involvement; and stage D, extension beyond the ureter to neighboring structures, adjoining lymph nodes or distant metastases. The significant of stage and grade appears to be similar to that in pelvic tumors.

Treatment

The treatment of urothelial tumors of the upper urinary tract remains basically surgical. Treatment strategy is dictated by detailed knowledge of the natural history of the disease, accurate staging and the experience of the individual surgeon.

It should always be considered that the multiplicity of urothelial tumors and the synchronous, asynchronous or metachronous character of the majority of the lesions can easily be characterized as a true neoplastic diathesis of the entire urothelium. Nonetheless, the prognostic significance of the tumor stage and grade has been stressed in several studies (Grabstald et al. 1971; Johansson et al. 1976) as well as the importance of any underlying disease, particularly 'Balkan' nephropathy (Petkovic 1975) and phenacetin abuse (Johansson et al. 1974; Johansson et al. 1976).

Total nephroureterectomy with or without excision of a periureteric cuff of the bladder has traditionally been the surgical procedure of choice for the majority of the renal pelvic tumors. However, more conservative surgery, i.e., nephrectomy and partial ureterectomy, has given good results in group I (benign papillomas) patients (Grabstald et al. 1971), as well as in rare cases of simultaneous bilateral neoplasms, 'Balkan' nephropathy or solitary kidney, when local excision is mandatory for the preservation of renal function (Johansson et al. 1974). It should be noted, though, that ureteric stump recurrences are not uncommon and frequently are associated with higher stage and grade tumors (Johansson et al. 1974). The role of lymph node dissection remains controversial and the overall 5-year survival for all grades is 44% (Ochsner et al. 1974) and for all stages 38% (Batata and Grabstald 1976). Radiation therapy has been disappointing in the management of upper urothelial tumors. Chemotherapy on the other hand still remains mostly experimental and no valid conclusions can be drawn from the very few case reports. The most promising agents are cisplatinum, vinblastine (Eyben et al. 1979), neocarzinostatin (Sakamoto et al. 1978), doxorubicin, and cyclophosphamide. (For additional details see 'Bladder Cancer', Chap. 5).

Sternberg et al. (1977) reported two patients suffering from metastatic transitional cell carcinoma of the renal pelvis who were treated with a combination of cisplatinum, cyclophosphamide and doxorubicin (CISCA). One had a partial remission of 1.5 months' duration and in the other two patients, stabilization of the disease for 6 and 2 months respectively was observed. In the same report two additional patients treated with a combination of doxorubicin and 5-fluorouracil were mentioned. Both died of progressive disease 2 and 2.5 months after beginning chemotherapy.

The same basic principles of therapy can be applied to ureteric cancer; the 5-year survival by stage is as follows: stage A, 90%; stage B, 43%; stage C, 16% and stage D, no survivors (Batata and Grabstald 1976; Ochsner et al. 1974). However, knowing the functional and pathophysiologic similarities to bladder cancer, it is reasonable to assume that preoperative irradiation could be of benefit in patients with advanced stage disease, and rare long-term survivors have been reported (Batata et al. 1975).

Local excision from its base is advocated for all benign polypoid lesions.

Follow-up

Because of the neoplastic potential of the entire urothelium, careful follow-up including detailed physical examination, urinalysis, cystoscopy and urine cytology at frequent intervals is advocated. However, the frequency, extent and duration of the follow-up still remain debatable (Gittes 1978).

References

Armstrong B, Garrod A, Doll R (1976) A retrospective study of renal cancer with special reference to coffee and animal protein consumption. Br J Cancer 33: 127–136

Batata M, Grabstald H (1976) Upper urinary tract urothelial tumours. Urol Clin North Am 3: 79–86

Batata MA, Whitmore WF, Hilaris BS, Tokita N, Grabstald H (1975) Primary carcinoma of the ureter. A prognostic study. Cancer 35: 1626–1632

Bloom NA, Vidone RA, Lytton B (1970) Primary carcinoma of the ureter. A report of 102 new cases. J Urol 103: 590

Boijsen E (1962) Angiographic diagnosis of ureteric carcinoma. Acta Radiol 57: 172

Donnelly DJ, Koontz WW (1975) Carcinoma of the renal pelvis: A ten-year review. South Med J 68: 943–946

Eriksson O, Johanssen S (1976) Urothelial neoplasms of the upper urinary tract. A correlation between cytologic and histologic findings in 43 patients with urothelial neoplasms of the renal pelvis and ureter. Acta Cytol (Baltimore) 20: 20–25

Eyben VF, Mattson W, Glifberg I, Lindholm CE (1979) Chemotherapy of advanced transitional cell carcinoma of the renal pelvis: Report of 3 cases treated with vinblastine and chlorethyl-cyclohexyl-nitrosourea. J Urol 121: 367–368

Ghazi RH, Morales AP, Al-Askari S (1979) Primary carcinoma of ureter. Report of 27 new cases. Urology 14: 18–21

Gittes RF (1978) Tumours of the ureter and renal pelvis. In: Campbell's Urology, vol II. Saunders, Philadelphia London Toronto, pp 1010–1032

Grabstald H, Whitmore WF, Melamed M (1971) Renal pelvis tumours. JAMA 218: 845–854

Johansson S, Angervall L, Bengtsson V, Wahlquist L (1974) Uroepithelial tumours of the renal pelvis associated with abuse of phenacetin-containing analgesics. Cancer 33: 743–753

Johnansson S, Angervall L, Bengtsson V, Wahlquist L (1976) A clinicopathologic and prognostic study of epithelial tumours of the renal pelvis. Cancer 37: 1376–1383

Johansson S, Wahlquist L (1977) Tumours of urinary bladder and ureter associated with abuse of phenacetin-containing analgesics. Acta Pathol Microbiol Scand 85: 768–774

Johnson DE, DeBerardinis M, Ayala AG (1974) Transitional cell carcinoma of the renal pelvis: Radical or conservative surgical treatment. South Med J 67: 1183–1186

Khan AV, Farrow GM, Zincke H, Utz DC, Greene LF (1979) Primary carcinoma in situ of the ureter and renal pelvis. J Urol 121: 681–683

Lucke B, Schlumberger HG (1957) Tumours of the kidney, renal pelvis and ureter. Atlas of Tumor Pathology, sect 8, fasc 30. Armed Forces Institute of Pathology, Washington

Mandell J, Magee MC, Fried FA (1977) Hypercalcemia associated with urothelial neoplasms. J Urol 119: 844–845

Mazeman E (1976) Tumours of the upper urinary tract calyces, renal pelvis and ureter. Eur Urol 2: 120–128

Ochsner MG, Brannan W, Pond HS, Collins HT (1974) Transitional cell carcinoma of the renal pelvis and ureter. Urology 4: 392–396

Petkovic DS (1975) Epidemiology and treatment of renal pelvic and ureteral tumours. J Urol 114: 858–865

Pollen JJ, Levine E, Van Blerk PJP (1975) The angiographic evaluation of renal pelvic carcinoma. Br J Urol 47: 363–369

Quattlebaum MS (1968) Adenocarcinoma of the renal pelvis. J Urol 99: 384–386

Reece WR, Koontz WW (1975) Leukoplakia of the urinary tract: A review. J Urol 114: 165–171

Resseguie JL, Nobrega GM, Farrow JW, Timmons JW Jr, Worobec TG (1978) Epidemiology of renal and ureteral cancer in Rochester, Minnesota, 1950–1974, with special reference to clinical and pathologic features. Mayo Clin Proc 53: 503–510

Sakamato S, Ogata J, Ikegami K, Naeda H (1978) Effects of systemic administration of neocarzinostatin, a new protein antibiotic, on human bladder cancer. Cancer Treat Rep 62: 453–454

Schmauz R, Cole P (1974) Epidemiology of cancer of the renal pelvis and ureter. J Natl Cancer Inst 52: 1431–1434

Sternberg JJ, Bracken BR, Handel PB, Johnson DE (1977) Combination chemotherapy (CISCA) for advanced urinary tract carcinoma. JAMA 238: 2282–2287

Wagle GD, Moore HR, Murphy PG (1974) Primary carcinoma of the renal pelvis. Cancer 33: 1642–1648

Chapter 5

Intravesical Chemotherapy for Superficial Bladder Cancer

M. S. Soloway

Introduction

One of the major challenges facing the urologist dealing with patients with super-ficial bladder cancer is the high likelihood that each patient will develop a subsequent tumor despite complete resection of an initial tumor(s). This incidence ranges from 40%–70% and is consistent among several reported series (Greene et al. 1973; Lerman et al. 1970; Pyrah et al. 1964; Williams et al. 1977). Prior to a review of the current status of intravesical therapy, it will be helpful to review the pathology of superficial bladder cancer, critical factors in endoscopic management, and the current concepts regarding the etiology of the high incidence of subsequent tumors.

Pathology

Histology

Papillary Tumors

The term 'papilloma' indicates an exophytic tumor that has a thin fibrovascular core covered by transitional epithelium whose cytologic appearance is identical to that of normal urothelium. Such a tumor is rare and the term papilloma should be restricted only to those tumors that have this histological appearance.

The majority of urothelial tumors appear as exophytic neoplasms in which the cells are arranged on fibrovascular stalks. These papillary tumors usually are of low cytologic grade and are non-invasive when they first present, however they have a marked propensity for 'recurrence'. The biologic potential of these tumors is related to the severity of cellular atypia. There may be a mixture of cytologic grades (I to III) within each neoplasm.

Supported in part by Grants CA15934 and CA18643 from the National Institute of Health through the National Bladder Cancer Project.

Flat Lesions

In contrast to papillary tumors, flat or sessile neoplasms probably develop from a region of urothelial atypia or dysplasia without concomitant hyperplasia. In the absence of a stalk, it obviously is difficult to identify these lesions cystoscopically especially if they are of low cytologic grades. Experience with the natural history of these preneoplastic lesions is limited and their biologic behavior is, therefore, poorly understood. These flat areas of urothelium, e.g. dysplasia/atypia, which correspond by virtue of their cellular architecture to the grade I and grade II papillary tumors might logically be termed flat, transitional cell carcinoma grade I and II. However, the terms dysplasia or atypia are preferable until the true biologic nature of these lesions is better understood. Flat tumors of high cytologic grade (grade III) are either confined to the urothelium in which case the term carcinoma in situ (CIS) is used or they are invasive. Invasive tumors are usually endoscopically apparent, however tumors confined to the urothelium, i.e. CIS, are not always detectable by endoscopic examination.

Transitional cell carcinoma in situ is often multifocal. The cells lack an orderly progression from the basal layer to the surface. Nuclear pleomorphism is prominent and the nuclear to cytoplasmic ratio is high. Mitoses may be frequent. Conceptually it is felt that bladder carcinoma in situ is a developmental transition from epithelial atypia and may represent an early phase in the evolution of invasive carcinoma. It must be emphasized, however, that the natural history of this lesion is quite variable.

The two major classification systems used for staging of urothelial tumors are the one introduced by Jewett and Strong (1946) and subsequently modified by Marshall (1952) and the TNM system (Prout 1976, UICC 1978). Tumors confined to the epithelium are termed stage O in the first system. This corresponds to Ta and TIS in the latter nomenclature. The Jewett and Strong system did not subclassify patients with CIS. Stage A in the Jewett and Strong, Marshall system is equivalent to T1 indicating tumor invasion into the lamina propria. Stage B1 lesions are equivalent to T2 and indicate invasion of the superficial muscle. In a discussion of superficial bladder cancer and the use of intravesical chemotherapy, our comments will be limited to the stage O–A or TIS, Ta, T1 lesions.

Cytology

Monitoring of patients with a history of bladder cancer following initial therapy is performed by endoscopy, bladder biopsies, and urinary cytology. Bladder biopsies can provide accurate information on the grade and level of invasion and are valuable when identifiable lesions are endoscopically visible. This technique is subject to sampling error particularly in the evaluation of flat, non-invasive carcinoma. An obvious disadvantage in monitoring a patient with periodic biopsies is the necessity of an invasive procedure.

Exfoliative urinary cytology is a valuable adjunct to cystoscopy and biopsy. It is inexpensive, non-invasive and samples the entire urothelial surface. Since the accuracy of cytology is quite high with lesions of higher cytologic grade, it is particularly helpful in the detection of carcinoma in situ. A positive cytology in a patient with histologic grade I papillary bladder cancer might alert the urologist to be suspicious of a higher grade neoplasm since the cytologic features of grade I tumors differ only slightly from those of normal urothelial cells and thus usually are not identifiable on examination of the urine. A bladder washing obtained by barbotage of approximately 50 ml saline performed at the time of cystoscopy appears to improve the yield of evaluable cells for cytopathologic analysis.

Certain conditions make interpretation of exfoliative urinary cytology more difficult. Inflammation may cause marked morphologic alteration in the epithelial cells with cellular enlargement and nuclear prominence. The nuclei of these epithelial cells may be coarsely granulated and may even have nucleoli. These changes reflect cellular reaction to injury. The nuclei in these cells usually are regular, however, an important distinction from the neoplastic nuclei.

Other situations can lead to difficulty in interpretation of urinary cytology. Radiation therapy produces significant cellular enlargement with occasional nuclear hyperchromasia. Antineoplastic alkylating agents may also alter the urothelial architecture. Cyclophosphamide is a prime offender due to the intense interaction of metabolites of this drug with the urothelium. In high doses these metabolites produce epithelial necrosis which is followed by regeneration. These regenerating epithelial cells are abnormal and are characterized by nuclear enlargement and hyperchromasia. These cells when exfoliated may look quite similar to neoplastic cells.

Although intravesical chemotherapy can produce some cytologic changes in exfoliated urothelial cells the experienced cytopathologist can usually distinguish these effects from malignant cells. The clinician should always provide the pathologist with pertinent data related to prior therapy, e.g. intravesical chemotherapy and radiation.

Endoscopic Assessment and Initial Management

At the time of endoscopy the urologist should fill out a bladder diagram indicating the number and size of each identifiable neoplasm and the location of each in relation to anatomic landmarks such as the bladder neck, ureteric orifices, lateral walls, and the dome. The surgeon should indicate whether the tumors are papillary or sessile.

Suspicious areas of the urothelium should be biopsied with a cold-cup biopsy forceps to avoid cautery artifact. Each specimen should be submitted separately indicating the biopsy site. In addition to biopsies from suspicious areas, selected-site or random biopsies may be obtained to determine whether there are urothelial abnormalities in endoscopically normal-appearing areas of the bladder. Selected-site biopsies are usually obtained lateral to each ureteric orifice, in the posterior midline, and the dome. A biopsy from the prostatic urethra should be considered when tumors are located near the bladder neck or if there is multifocal carcinoma in situ.

The initial endoscopic management of superficial bladder tumors usually includes resection of all visible tumor, if possible. Although this usually requires regional or general anesthesia, fulguration of small papillary tumors with or without selected-site biopsies is increasingly being performed as an outpatient procedure using intravenous sedation and topical anesthesia. If there is any suspicion of muscle invasion or doubt about the completeness of tumor removal, the surgeon should submit a separate specimen from the base of the tumor. If, however, the urologist is confident that he is dealing with a superficial papillary lesion such a biopsy is not necessary. The base of the tumor and at least 5–10 mm of adjacent urothelium should be thoroughly fulgurated unless the proximity of the ureteric orifice prohibits this. Transurethral management of multiple tumors is a painstaking procedure. The urologist must pay particular attention to areas of the bladder notoriously difficult to visualize such as the anterior wall at the bladder neck.

Patient monitoring following initial tumor resection must be planned according to the needs of the individual. Cytoscopy should be performed every 3–4 months, however the necessity for mucosal biopsies will depend on the appearance of the urothelium and the type and extent of prior lesions. Another factor is the reliance the clinician has on the accuracy of urinary cytology. The cooperation of an experienced cytopathologist allows the urologist to decrease the number of random mucosal biopsies in the absence of an identifiable lesion. If the voided or cystoscopic urine and bladder washing fails to reveal tumor cells the clinician can be reasonably confident a significant tumor is not being missed since high grade cells should almost always be identified. A positive cytology, on the other hand, indicates the necessity to search for a tumor, e.g. random biopsies, intravenous urogram. As patients respond for longer periods to intravesical therapy it becomes almost impractical to continue to perform numerous biopsies; thus the critical role of cytology.

Prognosis Following Surgery

Papilloma

The survival of patients harboring a papilloma is equivalent to the life expectancy of the general population in the same age range, provided that carcinoma does not subsequently develop. In a survey of 125 patients, Lerman et al. (1970) documented a 9.6% incidence of subsequent carcinoma; 5.6% were invasive lesions.

Carcinoma

The 5-year survival of patients with superficial carcinoma also is quite good. High grade tumors and those with multiple lesions carry a worse prognosis than those with low grade, solitary tumors. Barnes et al. (1977) reported a 73% 5-year survival rate for patients with stage A tumors. Patients with grade I tumors had a higher survival rate, 81%, than patients with grade II tumors, 59%. Greene et al. (1973) reviewed 100 consecutive patients with grade I transitional carcinoma and observed a higher recurrence rate in patients with multiple tumors, 88%, than in patients with single tumors, 68%. Of the entire group 10% eventually developed tumors with muscle invasion. He also noted that patients with stage A lesions had a somewhat poorer prognosis than those whose tumors were confined to the epithelium.

MacKenzie et al. (1981) reviewed the records of 292 patients with superficial transitional cell carcinoma seen between 1962 and 1978. They included 21 patients with stage B1 lesions. Two hundred patients (68%) were stage O and 71 (24%) were stage A. One hundred and thirty-eight (47%) never developed a subsequent tumor. Of those that did develop a recurrence, 25% eventually developed invasive carcinoma. The number of 'recurrences' did not increase the risk of subsequent invasion. The factor most likely to predict a subsequent invasive tumor was the grade of the initial tumor.

Anderström et al. (1980) found that invasion into the lamina propria was an important prognostic indicator. They found a 98% survival rate in 78 patients with non-invasive lesions (grades I–III); only three patients died of bladder cancer. In contrast, the 5-year survival rate was 75% in 99 patients with stage A lesions (grades

II–IV); 24 patients died of bladder cancer in 5 years. Lymphatic invasion proved to be a particularly poor prognostic sign.

The National Bladder Cancer Collaborative Group A (1981) recently presented data from a surveillance study on the natural history of patients with transitional cell carcinoma limited to the bladder and initially treated only by endoscopic means. Fifty-one percent (139) of 274 patients developed a subsequent tumor despite the fact that 96% initially were felt to be tumor free. The median time to recurrence was 35 months. Important, however, was the relative lack of progression. Only 15 of 175 patients (11.7%) with initial Ta lesions developed invasive tumors (ten T1, five T2). Of 73 patients with initial T1 tumors, 21% progressed to T2+ disease.

Carcinoma In Situ

One of the most difficult dilemmas in dealing with patients with superficial bladder carcinoma is the management of carcinoma in situ. Although we have accumulated accurate data on the natural history of exophytic papillary tumors, grade I and II/stage O or A, we lack sufficient knowledge of the natural history of carcinoma in situ. The literature on this subject over the last 20 years indicates a gradual change in treatment philosophy. Until recently the prevailing opinion was that CIS would inexorably progress to invasive cancer and cystectomy should not be delayed. Emphasis is now being centered not only on the wide range of time until progression but also on the potential for some of the cases to remain confined to the epithelium. Reasons for this apparent change in philosophy regarding the management of CIS include the use of intensive intravesical chemotherapy and introduction of new drugs as well as the more frequent use of mucosal biopsies with the resultant earlier discovery of CIS. As biopsies and cytology are performed more readily in individuals with irritative symptoms or concomitant low grade tumors, CIS undoubtedly is being discovered earlier.

Tannenbaum and Romas (1978) retrospectively reviewed 140 cases of CIS with a follow-up period of 14–21 years. This series is unique since the initial diagnosis was CIS, i.e. no history of a prior tumor. Forty percent of these patients progressed to stage A or B1 disease within 4–6 years; 10% progressed to stage B2 or C. After a 10-year follow-up, 60% had stage A–B1, and 20% progressed to stage B2 or C. By 15–21 years, 40% of the patients had died of bladder cancer with the majority of the remainder progressing to stages B2–D. Although this series does not provide details of therapy it does suggest, until proven otherwise, that carcinoma in situ gradually progresses to invasive carcinoma.

Riddle et al. (1976) reviewed the course of 36 patients who initially presented only with CIS; 23 had severe irritative symptoms and multifocal disease. At the time of definitive treatment, invasion was noted in 18 of these patients. Thirteen patients presented with minimal symptoms and therapy consisted of intravesical instillation of ethoglucid and/or endoscopic management occasionally combined with radium needle insertion. None of these patients died during a follow-up of 6 years. This report underscores the variable natural history of CIS and the importance of individualized treatment. Patients with multifocal disease probably should be considered for intravesical chemotherapy and monitored at 2–3-month intervals with cytologic and endoscopic examinations with multiple biopsies. If intravesical chemotherapy does not improve the irritable symptoms which frequently occur and urinary cytology does not revert to normal, cystectomy should be considered.

The rationale for this approach is suggested by the Mayo Clinic experience. In their initial series 73% of the patients developed invasive disease and 57% died of bladder cancer within 5 years of therapy which initially consisted of endoscopic management (Utz et al. 1970). In their recent report, however, 14 patients were treated with intravesical thio-tepa and only one patient developed invasive carcinoma (Utz et al. 1980). One explanation for this difference might be the use of intravesical therapy but an alternative one is that the patients in the second series were identified much earlier in the natural history of the disease. Longer follow-up will provide the answer.

On gross examination, CIS usually has a granular appearance. It is often reddish and may be slightly raised. CIS is often multifocal, a fact which has been substantiated by careful histologic mapping of bladders removed both for superficial and invasive disease. The distal ureter may be involved in 60% and the proximal urethra in 40%.

Virtually all patients with CIS will shed abundant high-grade cells into the urine. The report by Farrow et al. (1977) illustrates the potential of cytology in early detection of CIS. They followed 203 patients with a 'false positive' urinary cytology. That is, the cytology showed high-grade tumor cells despite normal endoscopic examination. Malignant urothelial disease was subsequently documented in 190 of these cases. Often the diagnosis was made by random mucosal biopsies. The responsibility of closely monitoring a patient with carcinoma in situ by cytology, endoscopy, and biopsies may be compared to watching a time bomb gradually tick off seconds. Whether intravesical chemotherapy can dismantle the bomb or whether it acts only by turning the clock back is uncertain and long-term follow-up on a much larger number of patients than is currently available in the literature will be required.

High Incidence of Subsequent Tumors

Theoretically bladder tumors which arise subsequent to an initial endoscopic resection or fulguration should be divided into two categories: true *recurrences* of the initial neoplasm and new *occurrences*. Unfortunately the differentiation between these two possibilities usually cannot be determined and, thus, the term 'recurrence' is often used to designate tumors that appear after initial management.

New Occurrences

Melicow (1952) introduced the concept that progressive neoplastic alterations arising from multiple regions of the urothelium are the main factor responsible for the high incidence of subsequent tumors after initial management. Investigating bladders removed for invasive carcinoma, he detected various degrees of dysplasia and CIS in areas that had normal appearance on gross inspection. Others have confirmed these findings by multiple section mapping studies of bladders removed for invasive carcinoma (Cooper et al. 1973; Farrow et al. 1976; Koss et al. 1974; Soto et al. 1977). Approximately 80% of such bladders revealed carcinoma or carcinoma in situ in previously unsuspected areas. This suggests that similar mucosal alterations are responsible for most 'recurrences'.

Further evidence supporting this concept is derived from data obtained by selected-site or random mucosal biopsies obtained from areas that appeared endoscopically normal and obtained from patients with superficial tumors. A surprisingly high incidence of hyperplasia, dysplasia, carcinoma in situ, and even carcinoma has been observed (Wallace et al. 1979). Soloway et al. (1978) detected 46% atypia, 14% CIS, and 16% carcinoma when biopsies were performed every 3 months in patients with superficial bladder cancer independent of whether a tumor was visible at each endoscopic sitting. Subsequent monitoring of these patients demonstrated a higher recurrence rate, 38%, in patients who had abnormal mucosal lesions compared to 15% in those who had no such alterations at the biopsy site (Murphy et al. 1979).

Wolf and Hojgaard (1980) performed mucosal biopsies in a number of patients with superficial lesions and found that patients harboring grade I tumors did not have evidence of dysplasia. Ten percent of patients with non-invasive grade II lesions had dysplasia. Those with grade II lesions with basement membrane invasion had a 62% incidence of dysplasia. The overall incidence of abnormal mucosal biopsies in the entire series was 54%.

Thus, bladder tumors developing from progressive growth in regions showing abnormal cellular architecture should be termed new occurrences rather than recurrences since they do not represent regrowth of the original tumor.

Evidence implicating known or suspected carcinogens in the etiology of bladder cancer supports the concept of diffuse urothelial neoplastic changes. Carcinogens present in the urine obviously are in contact with a major portion of the urothelium and would be expected to induce tumors in multiple sites over variable periods of time.

Tumor Implantation

A contributing factor to the high incidence of subsequent tumors may be the implantation or seeding of tumor cells on the urothelial surface during or following local resection or fulguration. Although current techniques are incapable of proving that implantation occurs in humans, experimental studies in animals and circumstantial evidence in man have led to growing evidence that implantation is a factor in the recurrence rate.

In an effort to simulate the clinical situation, Soloway and Masters (1980) devised a technique to cauterize a portion of the mouse bladder. Following fulguration transplantable transitional tumor cells were instilled into the bladder through a small urethral catheter. After 4 weeks, 54% of the cauterized bladders contained a tumor in contrast to only 12% in a comparable group of mice receiving an identical number of tumor cells but not preceded by fulguration. In humans, tumor cells regularly exfoliate from the transitional cell carcinoma, and it is reasonable to assume that the urothelial surface traumatized by instrumentation or resection might provide a fertile surface for these cells to implant.

Albarran and Imbert (1903) commented on the likelihood of implantation by noting the frequency of tumors in the ureter or bladder in patients with papillary tumors of the ipsilateral renal pelvis. Hollands (1950) believed that implantation was the likely explanation for the 3% incidence of tumors observed in the posterior urethra in patients developing a subsequent tumor since primary tumors at this site are quite uncommon, 0.5%. Many urologists can cite their personal observations on the frequency of subsequent tumors at sites not typical for initial tumors and potentially related to endoscopic trauma.

Boyd and Burnand (1974) carefully mapped the sites of initial tumors and compared this to the location of subsequent tumors. Only two of 32 patients, 6.3%, had primary tumors located on the vault whereas this site was the location of a subsequent tumor in 29 patients, 91%. Page et al. (1978) also showed a striking difference in the distribution within the bladder of primary and recurrent tumors. Concluding that implantation contributed to vault recurrences, Burnand et al. (1976) instilled 90 mg of thio-tepa into the bladders of 19 patients immediately after tumor resection in an attempt to eradicate any viable cells remaining in the bladder. A control group of 32 patients was treated by fulguration and resection alone. After 1 year there was a significantly higher incidence, 31/32, of recurrences in the control group compared to those receiving thio-tepa, 11/19, $P < 0.001$.

Possible evidence implicating endoscopic trauma in implantation and recurrences might be derived from the work of Van der Werf-Messing (1969). She and her colleagues manage most large superficial bladder tumors by suprapubic transvesical implantation of radium seeds. The recurrence rate using this technique is only 12.5% in a series of patients with T1 lesions. This is, of course, dramatically lower than the reported incidence following transurethral resection. Although radium seeds may eradicate preneoplastic cells or unrecognized tumors in sites distant from the primary tumor, it is possible that an alternative explanation is the avoidance of endoscopic trauma to the urothelial surface.

Intravesical Chemotherapeutic Agents

Since both multifocal field changes and implantation might contribute to the high incidence of subsequent tumors, it seems futile to rely solely on transurethral resection for the long-term management of superficial bladder cancer. Topical chemotherapy begun shortly after surgical resection might reduce the likelihood of true recurrences by eradicating viable tumor cells remaining in contact with the urothelium and might also diminish the number or frequency of new occurrences by exerting a cytotoxic action on the microscopic foci of carcinoma or CIS. Intravesical instillation of antitumor drugs exposes neoplastic cells to a relatively high concentration while minimizing systemic toxicity.

There is a need to standardize the definition of failure of a drug used for intravesical chemotherapy. With the introduction of more agents patients will increasingly be seen with superficial lesions after having received one or more doses of a drug. They may have received this drug in an attempt to eradicate a tumor, i.e. no concomitant endoscopic resection was attempted. This would be considered 'ablative' or 'definitive' therapy. Alternatively, the patient may have received 'prophylactic' therapy after endoscopic resection or fulguration of all visible disease.

Definitions of drug failure in these circumstances have been proposed by the National Bladder Cancer Collaborative Group A protocol committee. When used for ablative therapy the drug has failed if the tumor remains after a minimum of four instillations over a 3-month period. Another definition of failure includes tumor recurrence on maintenance intravesical chemotherapy despite initial successful tumor eradication by the drug. A third definition of failure is the development of a subsequent tumor while receiving regular, usually monthly, prophylaxis following initial tumor resection of fulguration.

Thio-Tepa (Triethylene Thiophosphoramide)

Since its introduction in 1961, thio-tepa (N,N',N''-triethylene thiophosphoramide) has been the drug most frequently used for intravesical chemotherapy of bladder cancer. This polyfunctional alkylating agent has been evaluated both for definitive therapy of existing tumors and for prophylaxis following endoscopic resection.

The overall response rate, complete and partial, when used for definitive therapy of low grade superficial tumors ranges from 47 to 79% (Table 5.1). The usual dosage

Table 5.1. Definitive therapy with thio-tepa for superficial bladder tumors

Authors	No. of patients	Complete response (%)	Partial response (%)	Failure (%)
Veenema et al. (1962)	16	25	38	18
Abbassian and Wallace (1966)	13	23	38	38
Edsmyr and Bowman (1970)	29	41	38	17
Pavone-Macaluso (1971)	25	32	32	36
Koontz et al. (1981)	95	23	24	39[a]

[a] Response of 12 patients (14%) unknown; if these are excluded, the combined response rate is 54%.

schedule consists of four weekly instillations of 30–60 mg diluted with 30–60 ml sterile water, followed by monthly administration of the same doses. The drug is usually instilled into the empty bladder and the patient should refrain from liquids for the previous 12 h. The recommended contact time is 2 h. Since myelosuppression is the major side effect of thio-tepa, leukocyte and platelet counts should be obtained before each treatment. Therapy should be withheld if the leukocyte count falls below 3500 and the platelet count drops below $100000/mm^3$.

In reviewing the studies on definitive therapy of bladder tumors with thio-tepa, there is an unfortunate lack of long-term follow-up. Thus, there is a paucity of data to allow objective determination of the need for long-term maintenance to prevent subsequent tumors. My current philosophy is to continue the drug on a monthly schedule for 1 year following either complete eradication by thio-tepa or a significant reduction in the number of tumors allowing endoscopic resection.

Our laboratory has carried out a series of experiments using an animal model which allows one to avoid the uncontrolled variability inherent in human studies and permit the examination of the entire bladder following thio-tepa instillation with comparison of the histology with urinary cytology in an attempt to find morphologic alterations induced by thio-tepa. The initial study analyzed the effect of thio-tepa versus saline on normal murine urothelium (Murphy et al. 1977). Evaluating both cytology and histology, no consistent morphologic differences were encountered between the treatment and control groups. There was a noted absence of atypical cells which usually are described in association with radiation or cyclophosphamide therapy. Thus, the appearance of malignant cytologic features from patients treated with thio-tepa should not be ascribed to a 'thio-tepa effect' but should be attributed to a malignant process. A subsequent series of studies evaluated the effect of thio-tepa on the induction of urothelial tumors by the carcinogen N-[4-(5-nitro-2-furyl)-2-thiazolyl] formamide (FANFT) (Murphy et al. 1978; Murphy and Soloway 1980). Thio-tepa or saline was introduced when the animals were known to have either atypia or carcinoma in situ. Following 3 weeks of therapy prominent cellular degeneration and vacuolation were observed and were believed to represent toxic effects of therapy. These effects were observed in the saline treated control animals, but were more prominent in those treated with thio-tepa. Nuclear changes, however, which might reflect alterations of cellular metabolism were uncommon. There was no statistically significant difference in the frequency of tumors between the treated and control animals. When thio-tepa was initiated at the atypia or CIS stage, there were significantly less high grade, high stage tumors in the thio-tepa treated group compared to the controls. This finding does suggest that thio-tepa retarded the progression of neoplasms from low grade, non-invasive lesions to high grade, invasive lesions.

If these animal studies provide an accurate indication of the effect of thio-tepa on human neoplastic urothelium, it may cause denudation of papillary growth with sloughing or flattening of the resulting naked fibrovascular stalks rendering them endoscopically invisible. Thus, the therapeutic effect will be recorded as a complete response although basal cells may not be entirely eradicated. Given sufficient time the tumor may reappear. This hypothesis does not negate the beneficial effects of thio-tepa. The drug may spare the patient repeated endoscopic sessions for fulguration of low grade tumors and its toxic effect may be sufficient to prevent implantation of tumor cells. Thio-tepa may also prevent the progression of low grade, non-invasive lesions to higher grade invasive tumors.

Several studies have now documented benefit from thio-tepa when used for prophylaxis, i.e. intravesical chemotherapy following complete visual eradication of all tumor (Table 5.2). The dosage, administration schedule, and the delay from resection to initiation of therapy varied widely in these studies. The amount of drug absorbed from the bladder depends on a number of factors including the intactness of the epithelium, presence of inflammation, the dose, and the duration of contact with the urothelium. When thio-tepa is instilled within 48 h following resection of a large tumor up to 60% of the drug may be absorbed (Pavone-Macaluso et al. 1976). Concern for myelosuppression has been the primary reason for delay in initiation of therapy following resection.

Table 5.2. Incidence of recurrence in patients treated with thio-tepa following surgery compared to surgery alone

Authors	Thio-tepa group		Control group	
	No. of patients	Recurrence rate (%)	No. of patients	Recurrence rate (%)
Burnand et al. (1976)	19[a]	58	32	97
Koontz et al. (1981)	45	40	47	60
Byar et al. (1977)	38	47	48	60
Schulman et al. (1979)	75	49	69	52

[a] Single dose.

Burnand and associates (1976) found minimal side effects following the instillation of a single 90 mg dose of thio-tepa immediately post resection. The drug remained in the bladder for 30 min. Gavrell et al. (1978) used 30 mg beginning immediately after surgery and continuing the drug twice daily for 3 days or weekly for 6 weeks. Both of these studies showed a significant reduction in the subsequent rate of tumors.

The National Bladder Cancer Clinical Collaborative Group compared the effects of prophylactic thio-tepa in 30 and 60 mg doses after resection of all visible tumor to a group not receiving chemotherapy (Koontz et al. 1981). Therapy was begun one month following resection. At 12 months, 66% of those receiving thio-tepa compared to 40% in the control group were free of tumor. This was a statistically significant difference, $P = 0.02$. There was no difference between those receiving 30 or 60 mg.

The EORTC Genito-Urinary Tract Cancer Cooperative Group compared the disease-free interval following transurethral resection of a superficial bladder tumor (Schulman et al. 1979). Patients received either thio-tepa 30 mg/30 ml, epipodophyllotoxin (VM-26), 50 mg/30 ml, or no therapy. Once again therapy was begun 1 month after surgery and continued weekly for 4 weeks and then monthly for 11 months. The recurrence rate was 49.3% in the thio-tepa group, 62.0% in the VM-26 group, and 52.2% in the control group. There was no significant difference among the treatment regimens. The recurrence rates per 100 patient months of follow-up were 6.93% for thio-tepa, 10.12% for VM-26, and 9.97% for the controls. Statistical analysis revealed a lower recurrence rate for the thio-tepa group than for VM-26 ($P = 0.03$) and for the control group ($P = 0.04$).

Mukamel et al. (1980) reviewed their experience with prophylactic thio-tepa. The first group of patients included 23 who had been treated by transurethral resection alone. Topical thio-tepa was instilled because of frequent recurrences. Patients in this group served as their own controls. A second group, 22 patients, received thio-tepa after their first transurethral resection and were compared to 19 patients who received only surgical therapy. The initial dose of thio-tepa, 15 mg in 60 ml water, was 7–10 days after tumor resection. The dose was increased by 15 mg weekly to a maximum of 60 mg. If the 60 mg dose was tolerated, this dose was instilled weekly for 5 weeks and then monthly.

Patients in group 1 averaged one recurrence per 11 months before thio-tepa. Following thio-tepa, the recurrence rate diminished to one tumor per 28.6 months. The patients in group 2 had one recurrence per 34.6 months compared to the control group who had one recurrence per 11.6 months. Initiation of intravesical instillation within 7–10 days after tumor resection did not produce significant side effects. Transient thrombocytopenia occurred in four patients and was easily controlled by cessation of therapy for 2–3 weeks.

England et al. (1981) used thio-tepa following endoscopic resection of multiple tumors in 40 patients. All patients had recurrent tumors. Twenty-seven patients had grade I and 13, grade II lesions. All of the patients with grade II tumors had lamina propria involvement.

Intravesical chemotherapy consisted of 30 mg thio-tepa for 2 h on postoperative days 1, 3, and 5. If myelosuppression occurred the dose was reduced to 15 mg.

These authors considered patients to have responded if there was no recurrence or if the number of new tumors was reduced to a small fraction of the established previous pattern. Following thio-tepa prophylaxis, 31 (78%) of the treated patients responded. Twenty-six became tumor free after one to three courses of thio-tepa. The remaining five responded as a result of the reduction of new recurrences to three or less. Nine patients failed to respond (22%) and two subsequently died from bladder cancer. There was no difference in the response rate between patients with grade I or grade II tumors. Of the 13 patients with grade II, stage T1 lesions, only two failed to respond to thio-tepa prophylaxis.

Eight of the 31 responders, 26%, have remained tumor-free without thio-tepa maintenance. Three of the entire group of patients died from bladder cancer during the follow-up period. Twenty-two other responders have required maintenance therapy.

Patients responding to thio-tepa usually respond after the first course of intra-vesical therapy. A common pattern was a reduction in the number of subsequent tumors with eventual clearance by endoscopic examination and selected-site or random biopsies. If responders subsequently developed another tumor after intra-vesical thio-tepa had been stopped or the intervals between the treatments markedly lengthened they usually would respond once again when thio-tepa was reinstituted.

Of the nine non-responders, four underwent progression with invasion of the muscle or a change in grade to grade III or both. The time interval between presentation and progression of the disease was 9 months to 6 years. Two other non-responders did not have tumor progression in the bladder but developed tumors of the upper urinary tract. The remaining three non-responders demonstrated no change in disease status 1½–2 years after thio-tepa was begun and 4–10 years after initial presentation.

Complications related to thio-tepa therapy were minimal. Irritative bladder symptoms did not occur and treatment was not interrupted due to myelosuppression.

Since I am concerned that implantation is a factor in the recurrence rate it is my preference to begin therapy as soon as feasible after a TUR. If the resection/fulguration is not extensive and the patient is younger than 70 years, I instill 60 mg thio-tepa diluted in 60 ml sterile water for 2 h the day after resection. Patients older than 70 years receive 30–45 mg. When an extensive resection is performed the initial instillation may be delayed for 3–5 days. Assuming that no significant myelosuppression occurs therapy is then continued weekly for 4 weeks and then monthly.

Ethoglucid

Ethoglucid (triethylene glycol diglycidyl ether) or Epodyl has been used for intravesical chemotherapy primarily in Great Britain. The effectiveness of this agent is equivalent to thio-tepa (Table 5.3), however the toxicity is reported to be less. The molecular weight of Epodyl is higher than that of thio-tepa, 252 versus 189, and this might account for the lower absorption rate.

Table 5.3. Response to ethoglucid in superficial bladder cancer

Authors	No. of patients	Complete response (%)	Partial response (%)
Colleen et al. (1980)	39	59	
Nielsen and Thybo (1979)	29	55	10
Robinson et al. (1977)	51	33	39

Robinson et al. (1977) observed 17 complete responses, 33%, and 20 partial responses, 39%, in a series of 51 patients treated with weekly therapy. Treatment-associated complications were minor with myelosuppression in only two patients.

Nielsen and Thybo (1979) reported a 55% complete response rate to ethoglucid among 29 patients with non-invasive papillary tumors who completed 12 months of therapy. Fifteen of the original 44 patients did not complete the study. There were three partial and 16 complete responses in the 44 patients, or an overall response rate of 43%.

Colleen et al. (1980) reviewed their experience with ethoglucid in 39 patients with well differentiated, non-invasive tumors. One hundred ml of a 1% ethoglucid solution was instilled weekly for 12 weeks, every other week for 3 months, monthly for 3 months, and once every third month thereafter. After 6 months of therapy 23 patients were disease free. The drug was stopped in ten patients because of cystitis. Among 11 patients who continued therapy, nine remained tumor free for 18–60 months, mean 37 months.

Riddle et al. (1981) reviewed the response of 139 patients to ethoglucid. These patients were treated between 1968 and 1978. All had multifocal superficial bladder tumors not amenable to endoscopic resection. The overall response rates showed minimal variation among patients with non-invasive papillary carcinoma compared to patients with tumors infiltrating the lamina propria. The long-term survival was quite different between these two groups. Fifty-one patients with non-invasive lesions had a 5-year survival rate of 73% in contrast to the 5-year survival of ten patients with T1 lesions, which was only 50%. Twenty-six percent of patients with initial TIS, Ta tumors were free of disease at 5 years compared to 13% with T1 lesions. Patients stopping therapy after 1 year and not going on the usual maintenance program usually developed a subsequent tumor.

Side effects related to ethoglucid occurred in 16% of the patients. Two developed a skin reaction; irritative symptoms were the predominant toxicity in the remainder.

Fitzpatrick et al. (1979) also reviewed a group of patients treated with ethoglucid. Complete remissions with multifocal TIS or T1 tumors occurred only if there was no lamina propria invasion. Only 30% of the initial group remained free of recurrence 5 years after beginning therapy. Failure to respond within 12 months, progression of tumor grade and progression from TIS to invasion were poor prognostic signs indicating the need for immediate cystectomy.

Thus, the two alkylating agents thio-tepa and ethoglucid appear to be roughly equivalent in efficacy and probably toxicity although occasional mild leukopenia and/or thrombocytopenia is more likely with thio-tepa. A prospective study comparing these relatively inexpensive drugs would probably be worthwhile but with the advent of newer drugs for intravesical therapy, which are potentially superior, this study may not be performed.

Doxorubicin Hydrochloride

Although doxorubicin (Adriamycin) has only recently been used for intravesical chemotherapy, a number of preliminary reports deal with the use of this agent for definitive therapy of superficial bladder cancer. Niijima (1979) reported a 56% complete plus partial response rate for a dose of 20 mg, 72% for 30 mg, and 74% for 50 mg instilled three times per week every 2 weeks.

Pavone-Macaluso (1979) evaluated 10, 20, or 40 mg doses on a weekly schedule for 4 weeks followed by monthly administration for definitive therapy. Although there were no complete responses, the partial response rates were 12.5%, 30%, and 33%, respectively. He also compiled data from several reports with a total of 98 patients. A complete response rate of 34% and a partial response rate of 43% were observed at doses ranging from 50–150 mg.

Edsmyr et al. (1979) used this drug on a slightly different schedule, 80 mg monthly. Patients had biopsy-documented TIS or T1 lesions. All eight patients with TIS receiving a minimum of five courses had negative endoscopic examinations and seven had a negative cytology. Patients with T1 lesions had a 50% (9/18) complete and 28% (5/18) partial response rate. There was no myelosuppression. Three patients had irritative symptoms related to therapy.

Jakse et al. (1981) treated 15 patients with carcinoma in situ. Nine had superficial bladder cancer at least 6 months before the diagnosis of CIS was established. Therapy consisted of either 40 mg in 20 ml saline (nine patients) or 80 mg in 40 ml (six patients). The lower dose was given biweekly and the higher dose monthly. Patients were monitored by mucosal biopsies as well as cytology. Tumor regression was observed in 10/15 patients (66%). The remission rate was the same at both dose levels. Only one of the five patients who did not show complete tumor resolution developed subsequent tumor progression. The follow-up, however, was only 6–22 months.

Severe cystitis was observed in four patients, one had severe hemorrhage after the initial instillation of the high dose doxorubicin.

Cytologic specimens obtained during the course of therapy revealed a gradual decrease in the number of cells obtained per specimen to about half of the initial value and this was a first indicator of tumor remission. The cytology correlated closely with the histologic findings. In no instance was CIS present when the cytology was negative.

The authors also monitored blood group isoantigens from the biopsy specimens. The blood group isoantigen was absent in CIS and all specimens showing atypia or normal urothelium had isoantigens present as indicated by the specific red cell adherence assay.

Jacobi et al. (1979) performed one of the few studies using doxorubicin for prophylaxis after endoscopic resection of all evident tumor. All patients had T1 lesions, grade I–II. Patients had an average of four prior transurethral resections. The dose was 40 mg/30 ml saline and therapy was given monthly. The mean follow-up was 22 months and ranged from 16 to 27 months. The average number of instillations was 14 with the mean total dose of doxorubicin being 560 mg. A control group did not receive intravesical therapy.

Only 5/15 patients treated with doxorubicin developed tumors in contrast to 13/15 control patients.

Schulman et al. (1981) recently completed a prophylaxis study using doxorubicin, 50 mg/50 ml. Intravesical therapy was begun within 24 h of transurethral resection of superficial tumors, stage O-A and repeated twice during the first week, weekly for 1 month, and then monthly for 1 year. Eighty-two patients had a one-year follow-up (23 primary tumors and 59 with recurrent lesions). Sixty-one percent were tumor free; 39% developed a recurrence. Only five patients had a more invasive recurrence. The recurrence rate was much lower in patients beginning therapy after their first tumor compared to those with prior recurrences, 17% vs 47%.

Although there was no systemic toxicity, 26% of patients had mild and 22% severe cystitis. The latter group could not continue on this regimen and were not included in the final analysis.

The overall incidence of recurrence at 1 year in this Belgian cooperative study does not differ from the prophylaxis study performed by the National Bladder Cancer Collaborative Group Study (Koontz et al. 1981) using thio-tepa despite the initiation of doxorubicin within 24 h and thio-tepa at 1 month. Once again a prospective randomized comparative trial for both definitive therapy and prophylaxis is needed.

Cis-Diamminedichloroplatinum (II) (DDP)

The impressive activity of DDP in advanced bladder cancer and an animal study indicating that intravesical administration can prevent tumor implantation in the FANFT-induced tumor model (Soloway and Masters 1980) suggest that DDP be evaluated for intravesical therapy in man. Only one clinical trial has been reported. Needles et al. (1981) treated 24 patients with CIS and/or T1 bladder tumors. Four patients received prior intravesical chemotherapy. Nine had CIS, seven T1 tumors, and eight both CIS and T1 lesions. Immediately before DDP, 18 patients had complete resection and an additional six partial resection of all observable lesions.

DDP was given weekly in a concentration of 1 mg/ml. Four patients received 50–150 mg and 20 received 100 mg. The median number of doses was 10 with a range of 3 to 19.

Tumor progression occurred in 21 of the 24 patients despite a median of 12 doses. One of these patients developed pulmonary metastases despite negative cystoscopic findings. The authors concluded that cis-platinum in the dose schedule used in the study was ineffective in controlling recurrent CIS and/or T1 bladder cancer.

Mitomycin C (MMC)

Mitomycin C is an antitumor antibiotic isolated from *Streptomyces caespitosus*. Its primary antitumor activity is via inhibition of desoxyribonucleic acid synthesis. The activity of mitomycin C in intravesical chemotherapy for superficial bladder cancer was initially evaluated in Japan. Mishina et al. (1975) treated 50 patients at a dose of 20 mg/20 ml sterile water, three times a week. Twenty-two patients (44%) achieved complete tumor regression and 16 patients (32%) had a partial remission. Twelve patients (24%) failed to respond to treatment. Mishina indicated that the response rates were directly related to tumor grade and size. Patients with low-grade (grades I and II) lesions had a higher response rate (89%) than patients with high grade (grades III and IV) tumors (36%).

Bracken et al. (1980) evaluated the effectiveness of intravesical MMC in 43 patients with stage O or A (TIS or T1) transitional cell carcinoma which was unsuitable for transurethral resection because of tumor location or the extent of tumor involvement. Patients were excluded if they had tumor invasion of the bladder muscle, white blood cell count below 3500/mm³, platelet count below 150000/mm³, or had been treated with other cytotoxic agents. Mitomycin C was administered in five dosage schedules: 20 mg/20 ml (10 patients); 25 mg/25 ml (11 patients); 30 mg/30 ml (6 patients); 40 mg/40 ml (6 patients); or 60 mg/30 ml (10 patients). The assigned dose was instilled in eight weekly courses. Patients were evaluated by endoscopy during the 11th week after therapy was started. The overall response rate was 84% (49% complete, 30% partial and 5% improved). Although the number of patients included in this study was not sufficient to permit definitive conclusions about the optimal dose, the response rate was higher with dosages above 25 mg.

I have treated 34 patients with superficial bladder cancer with MMC at the University of Tennessee Center for the Health Sciences. The results of the first 26 have been reported (Soloway et al. 1981a,b). Eight weekly doses of 30 mg/30 ml sterile water were administered to six patients and 28 received 40 mg/40 ml. Despite previous intravesical thio-tepa therapy, 24 patients had persistent tumors (Table 5.4). The ages of the 22 men and 12 women ranged from 49 to 97 years (mean 71 years). At least one tumor was histologically confirmed in each patient. A solitary lesion was not completely excised at the time of biopsy. All patients had one or more urothelial tumors at initiation of mitomycin C therapy. One patient had six papillary tumors scattered throughout the bladder, two had five lesions, and 31 had one to three endoscopically visible lesions. Six patients had multifocal carcinoma in situ. As indicated in Table 5.5, 12 patients had grade III tumors (CIS = grade III).

Patients were instructed to restrict their fluid intake for 10–12 h preceding MMC instillation. The catheter was removed following instillation and the patients instructed to void 2 h later. Therapy was repeated weekly for 8 weeks; 4 weeks later (week 12), response was evaluated by endoscopy and urinary cytology. The definition of complete response was related to the primary tumor type. The criteria for

Table 5.4. Mitomycin C therapy patient characteristics

Dosage	No. of patients	Average age	Range	Prior thio-tepa therapy No. of patients
30 mg	6	75	58–89	4
40 mg	28	67	49–97	20
	34	71		24

Table 5.5. Mitomycin C therapy: tumor characteristics

MMC Dosage	Grade/No. of patients			Stage/No. of patients	
	1	2	3[a]	O	A
30 mg	0	3	3	3	3
40 mg	7	12	9	19	9

[a] Includes CIS.

complete response of an exophytic tumor included the disappearance of all endoscopically visible lesions and negative urinary cytology. In patients with carcinoma in situ, complete response was based on random 'cold-cup' biopsy-proven absence of tumor and a negative urinary cytology. A partial response required more than a 50% reduction in the size of all tumors and the absence of new neoplasms. The majority of the complete responders continued to receive monthly mitomycin C therapy, with cystoscopic evaluation every 3 months.

Table 5.6. Results of mitomycin C therapy

Dosage	Complete response	Partial response	Failure	Total
30 mg	1 (17%)	3 (50%)	2 (33%)	6
40 mg	15 (54%)	9 (32%)	4 (14%)	28
	16 (47%)	12 (35%)	6 (18%)	34

The overall response rate was 82% (Table 5.6). No tumor was evident in 16 patients (47%); 12 patients (35%) achieved a partial remission. The response rate appeared to be somewhat better at the higher dose but the number receiving the 30 mg dose is too small to make any meaningful conclusion regarding the optimal dose. At the 12-week endoscopic session, complete necrosis of previous papillary tumors frequently was observed. Biopsy specimens usually cannot be taken from these firm areas due to the intense fibrotic response.

Although systemic mitomycin C is myelosuppressive, intravesical treatment did not result in leukocyte or platelet count reduction. This is consistent with the lack of absorption as indicated by serum samples obtained at various times after MMC instillation. This lack of absorption may be related to the molecular weight of mitomycin C (334) vs thio-tepa (189).

Side effects occurred in eight patients, all men, and consisted of moderate cystitis in four and drug-related desquamation of the palmar skin in four patients. In two patients the palmar desquamation was mild and subsided after treatment with hydrocortisone cream. In the other two the rash was severe and was accompanied by a macular rash in the perineal region with penile edema. One of these men responded to a topical steroid and diphenhydramine. This patient was instructed to thoroughly wash his hands and genitalia following each MMC instillation as well as the next several voidings. No new symptoms or rash appeared. The fourth patient did not respond to this regimen and MMC was discontinued.

We performed a series of patch and scratch tests on these patients with concurrent controls and believe that most of the cutaneous reactions are due to a contact dermatitis. Careful cleansing of the hands and perineum can prevent most of these reactions.

Experimental and clinical studies of mitomycin C have been conducted to evaluate the morphologic effect of the drug on murine and human bladder epithelium. Daskal et al. (1980) instilled mitomycin C in various concentrations into normal and tumor-bearing murine bladders. Two hours after instillation, the bladders were drained, excised and prepared for microscopic studies. Light microscopic examination demonstrated focal changes in both normal and tumor-bearing bladders treated with a dose of 5 mg mitomycin C. The normal bladders showed nuclear and cytoplasmic vacuolation, consistent with the onset of cell necrosis. The tumor-bearing bladders showed similar focal alterations. These effects were limited to epithelial cells.

The clinical and experimental studies by Murphy et al. (1981) focused on the drug-induced alterations that may mimic neoplasia and limit the efficacy of cytologic tests so helpful in patient monitoring. Drug-related changes that may be confused with malignant features were rare. Atypical cytologic changes found were confined to superficial cells.

Based on these results, the following conclusions were made: (1) Cellular abnormalities occurring after mitomycin C therapy were not drug-specific and were readily distinguishable from neoplastic changes; therefore, the drug will not limit the efficacy of urinary cytology in the follow-up of patients treated with MMC. (2) Prominent denudation, inflammation and edema detected in biopsy specimens of patients treated with mitomycin C correlated more with patterns of individual host response than with the dose or duration of therapy. (3) Fibrosis was rarely observed, indicating that scarring is not a predictable sequel of treatment.

Based on pilot series, mitomycin C may be the most active of the drugs currently under investigation. The low toxicity is a major advantage. A prospective trial comparing MMC with thio-tepa for definitive therapy of measurable superficial tumors is currently underway. Although the use of MMC for prophylaxis following transurethral resection has yet to be adequately studied there is little doubt that such a trial will be undertaken.

Bacillus Calmette Guerin (BCG)

The concept of using nonspecific immunotherapy for superficial bladder tumors is based on the assumption that there are specific antigens on the surface of bladder tumor cells and the contact between an immunostimulant, e.g. BCG, and the tumor may induce a more pronounced response to the tumor(s) than the patient was previously able to attain. Bubenik et al. (1970) identified tumor-specific antigens associated with transitional tumor cells. Some patients with urologic tumors, including bladder cancer, have impaired immunocompetence and the extent of disease correlates with the degree of immunocompetence. Investigation of the efficacy of immunotherapy in animal models has demonstrated that the success of immunostimulation in eradicating tumors is limited to a relatively small tumor burden. Thus, patients harboring small papillary tumors might be an ideal setting to test the effectiveness of nonspecific immunotherapy.

In other clinical and experimental tumor systems, the injection of BCG directly into a tumor is more effective than immunization at a distant site. When applied to bladder cancer the requirement of endoscopic injection might be a major deterrent. Injection of BCG directly into a tumor is not without risk. Side effects associated with intra-lesional BCG injection include: regional lymphadenitis, liver granulomas, and disseminated mycobacterial infection.

Another potential complication of nonspecific immunostimulation is the production of blocking antibodies with enhancement of tumor growth.

Martinez-Pineiro and Muntanola (1977) performed a small pilot study utilizing BCG in two different ways. Three patients with papillary tumors were treated by cutaneous scarification. Two additional patients with small papillary carcinomas had intra-lesional injection of BCG. The three patients in the first group had no response following scarification. Both of the patients having intra-lesional BCG showed significant tumor regression. One patient experienced a hypersensitivity reaction with fever, chills, and hypotension.

Martinez-Pineiro (1980) recently updated his experience with BCG. Twenty-nine patients were treated with prophylactic BCG, either by scarification alone, intra-vesical instillation alone, or a combination of the two. None of the 14 patients who started therapy after resection of their first tumor developed a recurrence; however 6 of the 15 (40%) with previous bladder tumors developed further neoplasms despite therapy. The overall recurrence rate was 20.6%. The authors felt that this compared favorably with recurrence rates following prophylaxis with thio-tepa.

The group receiving instillation alone had a lower recurrence rate than those receiving scarifications alone or instillation plus scarification. The authors mention that the group receiving instillations alone had a lower recurrence rate prior to entrance into the protocol than those in the other two groups.

Among the 19 patients receiving BCG instillations alone or in combination with intradermal scarification, 6 (31.5%) suffered cystitis; it was severe in 2.

Lamm et al. (1980) reported a relatively small prospective randomized study to compare standard endoscopic surgery for superficial bladder cancer to surgery plus BCG. All visible tumor was resected before BCG treatment. All patients in this study had bladder tumors resected within 3 years of entry. Thus, some patients had an interval in which they were tumor-free before entry to the study. Five patients with stage B tumors were included; four were randomized to receive BCG. A suspension containing 120 mg of BCG in 50 ml normal saline was instilled into the bladder and 5 mg (5×10^7 organisms) was given into alternate upper thighs using a Heaf gun weekly for 6 weeks beginning 1–2 weeks after transurethral resection of the tumor and/or at entry onto the protocol.

Side effects were minimal. Of the 18 patients receiving BCG, dysuria occurred in 17, urinary frequency in 15, and hematuria in 7. These symptoms usually occurred 1–2 days following intravesical therapy. Slight fever occurred in 4 patients and 4 had nausea and vomiting.

The rate of tumor recurrence was compared in the two groups. Eight of 19 control patients (42%) developed a recurrence with a total of 13 tumors. In the group receiving BCG, 3 of 18 patients (17%) had a tumor 'recurrence' with a total of six lesions.

The authors compared the incidence of recurrent tumors at matched intervals before and after entry onto the protocol. In the control group there was no change in the rate of tumor recurrence; patients receiving BCG experienced a statistically significant decrease in the incidence of tumors. The median time to recurrence was less than half in the control group compared to those receiving BCG.

Robinson et al. (1980) treated ten patients with recurrent T1 transitional cell tumors with intravesical BCG utilizing 1 ml Glaxo freeze-dried BCG vaccine weekly for 4 weeks and then monthly for 11 months. All patients had obvious tumor which was not resected at initiation of the study. Of the ten patients evaluable at the time of the report, two had complete tumor regression and an additional four had a partial response. Notably, two patients had systemic toxicity; one required antituberculous therapy.

Morales (1980) treated seven patients with carcinoma in situ with BCG. All patients had associated non-invasive papillary tumors which were fulgurated endoscopically but biopsies taken from other areas of the urothelium showed carcinoma in situ. BCG was administered weekly for 6 weeks by both intravesical instillation of 120 mg and intradermal injection of 5 mg. Eight weeks following the last immunization cystoscopic biopsies were obtained. Five of the seven patients were tumor free as determined by endoscopy, biopsies and urinary cytology. Follow-up ranged from 12 to 33 months, mean 22 months.

Endoscopy 8 weeks after completion of therapy showed variable degrees of inflammation in all cases. In only one patient was the endoscopic appearance suggestive of carcinoma; this was confirmed histologically. Biopsies always demonstrated a chronic inflammatory infiltrate suggestive of granulomatous reaction.

The evidence available from these small studies is insufficient to permit any firm conclusions regarding the place of BCG treatment in the management of superficial bladder tumors.

Perspectives

Several clinical trials using new drugs have justified the increasing incorporation of intravesical chemotherapy into therapeutic programs for bladder cancer patients. Until recently, thio-tepa and ethoglucid were the only agents used and they were largely reserved for patients unsuitable for surgery.

Treatment patterns are gradually changing on two levels. New agents such as mitomycin C and doxorubicin have been introduced. These drugs appear to produce higher objective response rates than thio-tepa, with less toxicity. Although a prospective randomized study has yet to prove their superiority the excellent response rates achieved in patients failing thio-tepa therapy and the impressive complete and partial regression rates documented by several investigators suggest this advantage.

Instillation of antitumor agents into the bladder within 48 h of complete endoscopic excision of superficial tumors has been shown to lengthen the tumor-free interval and reduce the recurrence rate. Although myelosuppression continues to be a therapy-associated risk when cytotoxic agents are instilled shortly after surgery, the degree of this effect seems to be correlated with the molecular weight of the agent. It is hoped that this potential hazard will be diminished or completely eliminated with the use of drugs that have a higher molecular weight than thio-tepa.

A number of aspects regarding the management of superficial bladder cancer with intravesical chemotherapy still need to be considered. More data on drug absorption are needed. The relative risks of local and systemic side effects for each drug need to be determined. Information must be gained on each drug's ability to enter normal or neoplastic urothelial cells. The role of urinary pH, bladder capacity, and vesicoureteric reflux, must all be correlated with toxicity and response rates for each drug. The duration of treatment has been largely empirical and limited to 1 or 2 h; varying this time may be fruitful. The frequency of instillation has also varied; however, most regimens rely on a weekly schedule. More frequent instillations might be more effective. The role of continuous bladder irrigation has not been explored. A low drug concentration in prolonged contact with the urothelium might provide superior cytotoxicity. The long-term side effects, e.g. carcinogenicity, must be addressed. This will probably necessitate work in an animal model since in the human it would be difficult to tell a carcinogen-related neoplasm from a subsequent new occurrence or true recurrence.

References

Abbassian A, Wallace DM (1966) Intracavitary chemotherapy of diffuse non-infiltrating papillary carcinoma of the bladder. J Urol 96: 461–465

Albarran J, Imbert L (1903) Les tumeurs du rein. Masson, Paris, pp 452–459

Anderström C, Johansson S, Nilsson S (1980) The significance of lamina propria invasion on the prognosis of patients with bladder tumors. J Urol 124: 23–26

Barnes RW, Dick AL, Hadley HL, Johnston OL (1977) Survival following transurethral resection of bladder carcinoma. Cancer Res 37: 2895–2897

Boyd PJR, Burnand KG (1974) Site of bladder tumour recurrence. Lancet II: 1290–1292

Bracken RB, Johnson DE, von Eschenback AC, Swanson DA, DeFuria MD, Crooke ST (1980) Role of intravesical mitomycin C in management of superficial bladder tumors. Urology 16: 11–15

Bubenik J, Perlmann P, Helmstein K, Moberger G (1970) Cellular and humoral immune responses to human urinary bladder carcinomas. In J Cancer 5: 310–319

Burnand KG, Boyd PJR, Mayo ME, Shuttleworth KED, Lloyd-Davies RW (1976) Single-dose intravesical thio-tepa as an adjuvant to cystodiathermy in the treatment of transitional cell bladder carcinoma. Br J Urol 48: 55–59

Byar D, Blackard C, Veterans Administration Cooperative Urological Research Group (1977) Comparisons of placebo, pyridoxine, and topical thio-tepa in preventing recurrence of stage I bladder cancer. Urology 10: 556–561

Colleen S, Ek A, Hellsten S, Lindholm CE (1980) Intravacitary epodyl for multiple, noninvasive, highly differentiated bladder tumours. Scand J Urol Nephrol 14: 43–45

Cooper PH, Waisman J, Johnston WH, Skinner DG (1973) Severe atypia of transitional epithelium and carcinoma of the urinary bladder. Cancer 31: 1055–1060

Daskal Y, Soloway MS, DeFuria MD, Crooke ST (1980) Morphological effects of mitomycin C administered intravesically to normal mice and mice with N-[4-(5-nitro-2-furyl)-2-thiazolyl] formamide-induced bladder neoplasms. Cancer Res 40: 261–267

Edsmyr F, Boman J (1970) Instillation of thio-tepa (tifosyl) in vesical papillomatosis. Acta Radiol [diagn] (Stockh) 9: 395–400

Edsmyr F, Berlin T, Boman J, Duchek N, Eposti PL, Gustafson H, Wilkstran H (1979) Intravesical therapy with adriamycin in patients with superficial bladder tumours. In: Montedison Läkermedel AB (ed) Diagnostics and treatment of superficial urinary bladder tumours. WHO Collaborating Center for Research and Treatment of Urinary Bladder Cancer, Stockholm, pp 45–54

England HF, Paris AMI, Blandy JP (1981) Intravesical thio-tepa as adjuvant to cystodiathermy in multiple recurrent superficial bladder tumours. In: Oliver RDS, Hendry WS, Bloom HJG (eds) Bladder cancer – Principles and combination therapy. Butterworths, London, pp 67–73

Farrow GM, Utz DC, Rife CC (1976) Morphological and clinical observations of patients with early bladder cancer treated with total cystectomy. Cancer Res 36: 2495–2501

Farrow GM, Utz DC, Rife CC, Greene LF (1977) Clinical observations on sixty-nine cases of in-situ carcinoma of the urinary bladder. Cancer Res 37: 2794–2798

Fitzpatrick JM, Khan O, Oliver RTD, Riddle PR (1979) Long-term follow up in patients with superficial bladder tumours treated with intravesical epodyl. Br J Urol 51: 545–548

Gavrell GJ, Lewis RW, Meehan WL, Leblanc GA (1978) Intravesical thio-tepa in the immediate post-operative period in patients with recurrent transitional cell carcinoma of the bladder. J Urol 120: 410–411

Greene LG, Hanash KA, Farrow GM (1973) Benign papilloma or papillary carcinoma of the bladder? J Urol 110: 205–207

Hollands FG (1950) The results of diathermy treatment of villous papilloma of the bladder. Br J Urol 22: 342–375

Jacobi GH, Kurth KH, Klippel KF, Hohenfellner R (1979) On the biological behaviour of T1-transitional cell tumours of the urinary bladder and initial results of the prophylactic use of topical adriamycin under controlled and randomized conditions. In: Montedison Läkermedel AB (ed) Diagnostics and treatment of superficial urinary bladder tumours. WHO Collaborating Center for Research and Treatment of Urinary Bladder Cancer, Stockholm, pp 83–94

Jakse G, Hofstadter F, Marberger H (1981) Intracavitary doxorubicin hydrochloride therapy for carcinoma in-situ of the bladder. J Urol 125: 185–190

Jewett HG, Strong GH (1946) Infiltrating carcinoma of the bladder: Relation of depth of penetration of the bladder wall to incidence of local extension and metastases. J Urol 55: 366–372

Koontz WW Jr, Prout GR Jr, Smith W, Frable WJ, Minnis JE (1981) Use of intravesical thio-tepa in management of non-invasive carcinoma of bladder. J Urol 125: 307–312

Koss LG, Tiamson EM, Robbins MA (1974) Mapping cancerous and precancerous bladder changes: A study of the urothelium in ten surgically removed bladders. JAMA 227: 281–286

Lamm DL, Thor DE, Harris SC, Rayna JA, Stogdill VD, Radwin HM (1980) Bacillus Calmette-Guérin immunotherapy of superficial bladder cancer. J Urol 124: 38–42

Lerman RI, Hutter RVP, Whitmore WF Jr (1970) Papilloma of the urinary bladder "Cancer 25: 333–342

MacKenzie N, Torti FM, Faysa L (1981) Natural history of superficial bladder tumors. Proc Am Assoc Cancer Res 22: 198

Marshall VF (1952) The relation of the preoperative estimate to the pathologic demonstration of the extent of vesical neoplasms. J Urol 68: 714–723

Martinez-Pineiro JA (1980) BCG vaccine in the treatment of non-infiltrating papillary tumours of the bladder. In: Pavone-Macaluso M, Smith PH, Edsmyr F (eds) Bladder tumors and other topics in urological oncology. Plenum Press, New York, pp 175–184

Martinez-Pineiro JA, Muntanola P (1977) Nonspecific immunotherapy with BCG vaccine in bladder tumors — a preliminary report. Eur Urol 3: 11–22

Melicow MM (1952) Histological study of vesical urothelium intervening between gross neoplasms in total cystectomy. J Urol 68: 261–279

Mishina T, Oda K, Murata S, Ooe H, Mori Y, Takahashi T (1975) Mitomycin C bladder instillation therapy for bladder tumors. J Urol 114: 217–219

Morales A (1980) Treatment of carcinoma in-situ of the bladder with BCG. A phase II trial. Cancer Immunol Immunoter 9: 69–72

Mukameol E, Zitron S, Nissenkorn I, Servadio C (1980) Prophylactic effect of triethylene thiphasphramide on the recurrence rate of superficial bladder tumors. Isr J Med Sci 16: 714–716

Murphy WM, Nagy GK, Rao MK, Soloway MS, Parija GC, Cox CE, Friedell GH (1979) 'Normal' urothelium in patients with bladder cancer. Cancer 44: 1050–1058

Murphy WM, Soloway MS, Lin CJ (1977) Morphologic effects of thio-tepa on mouse urothelium. Acta Cytol (Baltimore) 21: 701–704

Murphy WM, Soloway MS, Lin CJ (1978) Morphologic effects of thio-tepa on mammalian urothelium: Changes in abnormal cells. Acta Cytol (Baltimore) 22: 550–554

Murphy WM, Soloway MS (1980) The effect of thio-tepa on developing and established mammalian bladder tumors. Cancer 45: 870–875

Murphy WM, Soloway MS, Crabtree WM (1981) The morphologic effects of mitomycin C in mammalian urinary bladder. Cancer 47: 2567–2574

National Bladder Cancer Collaborative Group A, Heney NM, Ahmed S, Flanagan MJ, Frable J, Corder MP, Hafermann MD (1981) Superficial bladder cancer: Progression and recurrence. Presented at AUA Annual Meeting, May 10–14, Boston, Mass

Needles B, Blumenreich M, Yagoda A, Sogani P, Whitmore WF (1981) Intravesical cisplatin for superficial bladder cancer. Proc Am Assoc Cancer Res 22: 158, 625

Nielsen HV, Thybo E (1979) Epodyl treatment of bladder tumours. Scand J Urol Nephrol 13: 59–63

Niijima T (1979) Intravesical therapy with adriamycin and new trends in the diagnostics and therapy of superficial urinary bladder tumours. In: Montedison Làkermedel AB (ed) Diagnostics and treatment of superficial urinary bladder tumours. WHO Collaborating Center for Research and Treatment of Urinary Bladder Cancer, Stockholm, pp 37–44

Page BH, Levison VB, Curwen MP (1978) The site of recurrence of non-infiltrating bladder tumours. Br J Urol 50: 237–242

Pavone-Macaluso M (1971) Chemotherapy of vesical and prostatic tumours. Br J Urol 43: 701–708

Pavone-Macaluso M (1979) Intravesical treatment of superficial (T1) urinary bladder tumours: A review of 15-year experience. In: Montedison Läkermedel AB (ed) Diagnostics and treatment of superficial urinary bladder tumours. WHO Collaborating Center for Research and Treatment of Urinary Bladder Cancer, Stockholm, pp 21–36

Pavone-Macaluso M, Gebbia N, Biondo F, Bertolini S, Caramia G, Rizzo FP (1976) Permeability of the bladder mucosa to thio-tepa, adriamycin, and daunomycin in men and rabbits. Urol Res 4: 9–13

Prout GR Jr (1976) The surgical management of bladder carcinoma. Urol Clin North Am 3: 149–175

Pyrah LN, Raper FP, Thomas GM (1964) Report of a follow-up of papillary tumours of the bladder. Br J Urol 36: 14–25

Riddle PR, Chisholm GD, Trott PA, Pugh RCB (1976) Flat carcinoma in-situ of bladder. Br J Urol 47: 829–833

Riddle PR, Khan O, Fitzpatrick JM, Oliver RTD (1982) Prognostic factors influencing survival of patients receiving intravesical epodyl. J Urol 000: 000–000

Robinson MRG, Richards B, Adib R, Akdas A, Rigby CC, Pugh RCB (1980) Intravesical BCT (Bacillus Calmette-Guérin) in the management of T1, N^X, M^X transitional cell tumors in the bladder: A toxicity study. In: Pavone-Macaluso M, Smith PH, Edsmyr F (eds) Bladder tumors and other topics in urological oncology. Plenum Press, New York, pp 171–174

Robinson MRG, Shetty MB, Richard B, Bastable J, Glashan RW, Smith PH (1977) Intravesical epodyl in the management of bladder tumors: Combined experience of the Yorkshire Urological Cancer Research Group. J Urol 118: 972–973

Schulman CC, Denis LJ, Oosterlinck W, DeSy W, Chantrie M, Van Cangh J (1981) Early adjuvant adria-mycin in superficial bladder cancer. Presented at the AUA Annual Meeting, May 10–14, Boston, Mass

Schulman C, Sylvester R, Robinson M, Smith P, Lachand A, Denis L, Pavone-Macaluso M, DePauw M, Staquet M (1979) Adjuvant therapy of T1 bladder carcinoma: Preliminary results of an EORTC randomized study. Recent Results Cancer Res 68: 338–345

Soloway MS, Masters S (1980) Urothelial susceptibility to tumor cell implantation — influence of cauter-ization. Cancer 46: 1158–1163

Soloway MS, Murphy WM, DeFuria MD (1981a) Intravesical mitomycin C in superficial bladder cancer. Proc Am Soc Clin Oncol 22: 469

Soloway MS, Murphy WM, DeFuria MD, Crooke ST, Finebaum P (1981b) The effect of mitomycin C (MMC) on superficial bladder cancer. J Urol 125: 646–648

Soloway MS, Murphy WM, Rao MK, Cox CE (1978) Serial multiple-site biopsies in patients with bladder cancer. J Urol 120: 57–59

Soto EA, Friedell GH, Tiltman AJ (1977) Bladder cancer as seen in giant histologic sections. Cancer 39: 447–455

Tannenbaum M, Romas NA (1978) The pathobiology of early urothelial cancers. In: Skinner DG, DeKernion JB (eds) Genito-urinary cancer. Saunders, Philadelphia, pp 232–255

UICC (1978) TNM classification of malignant tumors, 3rd edn. International Union Against Cancer, Geneva

Utz DC, Farrow GM, Rife CC (1980) Carcinoma in-situ of the bladder. Cancer 45: 1842–1848

Utz DC, Hanash KA, Farrow GM (1970) The plight of the patients with carcinoma in-situ of the bladder. J Urol 103: 160

Van der Werf-Messing G (1969) Carcinoma of the bladder treated by suprapubic radium implants. Eur J Cancer 5: 277–285

Veenema RJ, Dean AL Jr, Roberts M, Fingerhurt B, Chowdhury BK, Tarassoly H (1962) Bladder carcinoma treated by direct instillation of thio-tepa. J Urol 88: 60–63

Wallace DMA, Hindmarsh JR, Webb JN, Busuttil A, Hargreave TB, Newsam JE, Chisholm GD (1979) The role of multiple mucosal biopsies in the management of patients with bladder cancer. Br J Urol 51: 535–540

Williams JL, Hammonds JC, Saunders N (1977) T1 bladder tumours. Br J Urol 49: 663–668

Wolf H, Hojgaard K (1980) Urothelial dysplasia in random mucosal biopsies from patients with bladder tumors. Scand J Urol Nephrol 14: 37–41

Chapter 6

Chemotherapy for Advanced Urothelial Tract Tumors

A. Yagoda

Introduction

There are approximately 30000 new cases of bladder cancer and 10000 deaths annually in the United States. Although bladder tumors occur in patients under the age of 50 years, the majority of cases are aged between 65 and 70. In the Western Hemisphere and Europe, bladder tumors are of the transitional cell (epidermoid) variety in over 95% of cases and only 3% are adenocarcinoma—mostly in the dome of the bladder and of urachal origin. In contrast, schistosomiasis-induced or bilharzial bladder cancer in Egypt and in India is of the squamous cell variety in over 75% of cases (Gad-el-Mawla et al. 1979). In the Western Hemisphere, a strong link to various chemical carcinogens as inciting or promoting agents has been firmly established (Cohen 1979) and it is therefore surprising that the incidence of bladder cancer has not increased significantly (thus far) in the United States during the past 10–20 years.

Presentation and Biological Behavior

Initially, patients often complain of hematuria, increased urinary frequency or pain with urination. Carefully executed urinary cytology (PAP test) will generally establish the diagnosis in well over 65% of cases (Farrow 1979). Patients with high grade (II, III) lesions or carcinoma-in-situ tend to have a much higher incidence of positive urinary PAPs compared to patients with grade I lesions. Cystoscopy and biopsy are always needed to establish the diagnosis. Patients who present with a single low grade lesion (many pathologists consider benign papilloma a grade I transitional cell carcinoma) have approximately a 30% chance of developing another lesion within 5 years, while those who present with two or more of these tumors have a 70% chance for tumor recurrence (Whitmore 1979). However, well over three-fourths of patients who present with carcinoma-in-situ eventually will develop invasive bladder cancer.

Carcinoma-in-situ as well as grades I–II superficial carcinomas have a tendency to recur both in time and space. This potential for multiplicity has been labelled 'polychronotropism'.

When tumors recur in large numbers and at frequent intervals, and cannot be adequately controlled with either transurethral resection or intravesical chemotherapy, radical cystectomy is generally recommended. The 5-year survival rate in this small group of patients is excellent — 90%–95%. Low grade tumors which invade lamina propria or half-way through the muscularis (stages A and B1, or T1 and T2) are treated, in most instances, by transurethral resection. Some urologists, however, prefer segmental resection for B1 lesions. If a high grade tumor is found, radical cystectomy or 'curative' radiation therapy (>5000–6000 rads) can be performed. In selected cases, particularly those with a single lesion without evidence of surrounding carcinoma-in-situ, segmental resection can also be curative (Whitmore 1979). For tumors which invade the deeper muscle layers of the bladder wall or which have extravesical extension (states B2 and C, or T3 and T4) radical cystectomy or 'curative' irradiation are the treatments of choice (Cummings et al. 1979).

Not infrequently, patients who have bladder tumors also exhibit carcinoma in situ in the urethra and ureter, and a radical cystectomy is combined with urethrectomy and partial ureterectomy (Schellhammer and Whitmore 1976). With the combination of preoperative irradiation and radical cystectomy, 5-year survival approaches 40%–50% in surgically staged and 30%–40% in clinically staged patients. However, when such therapy is performed in patients who have lymph node metastases, the 5-year survival rates are exceedingly poor — 0%–15%. In fact, only half of the patients who have palpable obturator, external iliac, or hypogastric lymph node involvement at surgery survive 10–14 months, and less than 15% survive 2 years regardless of the therapeutic approach. Without surgery, death is usually secondary to uremia, while after radical cystectomy and an ileal conduit, death generally is due to disseminated disease.

Topical Chemotherapy

The treatment of superficial carcinomas by repeated transurethral resection or by intravesical triethylene thiophosphoramide, mitomycin C, epodyl, adriamycin and more recently, BCG, remains in the hands of the urologist (Soloway and Murphy 1979). Recent randomized studies suggest that intravesical immunotherapy with BCG can control the number and frequency of local tumor recurrences, particularly for low grade, low stage lesions, and also that triethylene thiophosphoramide has some prophylactic benefit when initial lesions are destroyed completely with chemotherapy. In addition, a recent randomized study by Burnard et al. (1976) showed a decrease in the incidence of so-called 're-implantation' tumors when triethylene thiophosphoramide is used immediately after transurethral resection. Murphy and Soloway (1980) confirmed the efficacy of this agent in the prevention of re-implanation tumor recurrences in a bladder cancer model (FANFT) in mice. Intravesical chemotherapy is considered in detail in Chap. 5.

Systemic Chemotherapy

During the past 5 years chemotherapy has been recognized as an effective component in the treatment of advanced disseminated urothelial tract tumors (transitional cell carcinoma of the renal pelvis, ureter, bladder, urethra and prostatic ducts). Medical oncologists and urologists should be aware of the variety of drugs available and the future adjuvant role for chemotherapy in patients who are at risk of relapse after preoperative irradiation and surgery.

Single Agents

cis-Diamminedichloride platinum II, or cisplatin, is the most effective single agent in advanced urothelial tract tumors. Approximately one-third of patients will respond, and tumor regression is evident usually in 1–4 weeks after beginning therapy. In fact, almost all responses occur within two doses (4–6 weeks) of cisplatin (Yagoda et al. 1976; 1980). The most commonly employed dosage schedule is 70 mg/m^2 IV, every 3–4 weeks. Other schedules have been tried but there is no evidence indicating an enhanced response rate or remission duration with different schedules (Merrin 1979).

Table 6.1. Chemotherapy regimens for urothelial tract tumors

Drug(s)	Dosage and schedule
Cisplatin	70 mg/m^2 IV every 3–4 weeks
	20 mg/m^2 × 5 consecutive days IV every 3–4 weeks
Adriamycin	45–60–75 mg/m^2 IV every 3 weeks
Methotrexate	0.5–0.75–1.0 mg/kg IV every week
	100–200 mg IM – folinic acid rescue every 2 weeks
Mitomycin C	10–15–20 mg/m^2 IV every 6 weeks
Cyclophosphamide	1000 mg/m^2 IV every 3 weeks
Cisplatin	70 mg/m^2 IV every 3–4 weeks
+ adriamycin	30–45 mg/m^2
Cisplatin	70 mg/m^2
+ adriamycin	30–45 mg/m^2 IV every 4 weeks
+ cyclophosphamide	250–500 mg/m^2
Adriamycin	50–60 mg/m^2 IV every 3 weeks
+ 5-fluorouracil	500–600 mg/m^2

Table 6.2. Chemotherapy response rates in urothelial tract tumors

Drug(s)	% Response
Single agents	
Cisplatin	35
Methotrexate	28
Adriamycin	17
Mitomycin C	14
Neocarzinostatin	5–70
5-Fluorouracil	35 no disease-oriented trials
Bleomycin	5
VM-26	20
Combination regimens	
Cisplatin	
+ Adriamycin	42
+ Cyclophosphamide	38
+ Adriamycin + cyclophosphamide	41
+ Adriamycin + 5-fluorouracil	41
Adriamycin	
+ VM-26	17
+ Cyclophosphamide	18
+ 5-Fluorouracil	39

Unfortunately many patients with bladder cancer have had repeated episodes of urinary tract obstruction and chronic pyelonephritis and, thus, do not possess adequate renal function for this nephrotoxic drug. All patients must have a 24-h urinary creatinine clearance of >55–60 ml/min, or normal blood urea nitrogen and creatinine levels before starting cisplatin. Patients are hospitalized for 48–72 h in order to administer intravenous hydration sufficient to ensure a urinary output of approximately 100 ml/h for 4–6 h before and 10–12 h after cisplatin administration.

The average duration of response with cisplatin is only 5 months, but occasionally patients have had remissions persist for more than 12–48 months. Unmaintained remissions usually last no more than 3 months, but re-institution of cisplatin occasionally will induce a second remission. Responses occur in pulmonary, nodal, hepatic and intra-abdominal lesions — rarely in osseous metastases. Responders can be treated with cisplatin every 6–8 weeks, but if tumor recurs, the interval should be reduced to 3 weeks. Cisplatin does not enter the central nervous system and the drug is therefore useless for treating spinal cord or brain metastases. In addition, recent evidence suggests that cisplatin is marginally effective in controlling intravesical disease (Soloway 1978; Oliver 1980; Herr 1980).

Adriamycin has been studied extensively in patients with metastatic bladder cancer and the overall response rate is only 15%–20% (Yagoda et al. 1977b). Remission tends to occur during the second or third course and seems to be dose-related. Patients who receive 60 or 75 mg/m² every 3 weeks have a slightly higher response rate compared to those given 30–45 mg/m² (O'Bryan et al. 1977). Duration of response is only 3–4 months and complete and long-lasting remission is rare. The initial dose is 45 or 60 mg/m² IV every 3 weeks, with a 15 mg/m² increase in dosage as tolerated. White blood cell and platelet counts should be obtained 7–14 days after adriamycin in order to adjust doses appropriately.

Methotrexate, which has been evaluated in Europe and recently in the United States, also induces remission in about 25%–30% of cases (Hall et al. 1974; Turner et al. 1977; Yagoda et al. 1980; Natale et al. 1981). Response occurs rapidly, within 7–21 days, and is rare after 5 weeks of therapy. Many dosage schedules have been employed, but a simple, yet effective, schedule is 0.5, 0.75, 1.0, or 1.25 mg/kg IV, every 3 weeks. Adequate renal function is imperative and no folic acid should be taken concurrently. At Memorial Hospital, the use of probenecid (which can delay methotrexate excretion and enhance toxicity) and sulfatrimethoprim compounds (i.e. Septra, Bactrim) are avoided. The average duration of remission is 5 months, but some patients have achieved a complete remission for more than 20 months. Data recently presented by Oliver (1980) and Turner et al. (1977) indicate that methotrexate may be more active than cisplatin in treating intravesical and loco-regional disease.

Other doses and schedules have been employed (i.e., 50 mg p.o., every 1–2 weeks; 100 mg IM, every 1–2 weeks; and 200 mg IM, with citrovorum factor rescue every 1–2 weeks), but there has been no randomized trial documenting increased efficacy with higher doses (Natale et al. 1981). However, the Royal Marsden Group (Hall et al. 1974; Turner et al. 1977) described a higher response rate with higher doses. When larger doses of methotrexate are given, alkalinization of the urine should be attempted with orally or intravenously administered sodium bicarbonate.

Other chemotherapeutic agents have been studied in drug-oriented trials but rarely in disease-oriented phase II trials which attempt to define a clear end-point of response. Mitomycin C, an anti-tumor antibiotic, used in the treatment of patients with gastric or pancreatic cancers, has some efficacy against transitional cell carcinoma. In 1973, Early et al. reported responses in approximately 20% of patients. Of note, mitomycin C, 10–15 mg/m² IV, every 5–6 weeks, can be administered to patients with compromised renal function or with cardiac abnormalities. Dose adjustment is made on the basis of the white blood cell and platelet count nadirs 28 and 35 days after beginning therapy.

The podophyllin derivative, VM-26, has been evaluated in Europe and preliminary data suggest anti-tumor activity in bladder cancer (EORTC 1972; Pavone-Macaluso et al. 1976; Mechl et al. 1977). A new podophyllin derivative, VP-16, is under study (Nissen et al. 1980). Bleomycin has demonstrated no activity in this disease (Pavone-Malcaluso et al. 1976). While the data on a new anti-tumor antibiotic, neocarzino-statin, is limited, Natale et al. (1980) have found no anti-tumor activity in patients with disseminated disease compared to Sakamoto et al. (1978) who described good response rates with intravenous and intravesical administration in patients with intra-vesical low stage lesions. 5-Fluorouracil, which has been studied (Carter 1978) in many drug-oriented phase II trials in varying dosages and schedules, needs to be analyzed again with presently employed criteria for response. Although response rates as high as 30%–35% have been recorded, a recent trial by Duchek et al. (1980) found remissions in less than 10% of cases. At best, 5-fluorouracil should be considered a secondary drug for the treatment of urothelial tract tumors.

Combination Therapy

Many drug combinations have also been tried, mostly incorporating adriamycin or cisplatin (Yagoda 1980). While the combinations of adriamycin and cyclophos-phamide (Merrin et al. 1975; Yagoda et al. 1977a), or VM-26 (Rodriguez et al. 1977) appear to be no better than adriamycin used singly (Yagoda et al. 1977b), adriamycin, 50–60 mg/m^2, and 5-fluorouracil, 500–600 mg/m^2 (Cross et al. 1976; EORTC 1977; Al-Sarraf et al. 1977), have been reported to induce remissions in 30%–40% of cases. However, without randomized trials documenting the types of patients entered, lesions measured, and categories of response, the latter combination should be considered only as a potential 'backup' regimen.

Cisplatin induces remissions in 35% (57 of 162) of cases (Yagoda 1980). The 95% confidence limits (28%–43%) suggest that results of many cisplatin combination regimens could statistically be attributed to the efficacy of cisplatin alone. The current, prospectively randomized trials should answer the question whether cisplatin-containing regimens are truly more effective than cisplatin singly. Such trials in patients with bladder cancer are, at times, difficult to organize because of the lack of so called 'indicator' lesions i.e. bidimensionally measurable masses (Yagoda 1977). Recently, computerized (transaxial) tomography (CT) has enlarged the number of patients available for phase II trials. However, even by CT not all masses are truly bidimensionally measurable and accurate assessment may be extremely difficult, particularly after radiation fibrosis, a not infrequent occurrence after 5000–6500 rads. In a recent study at Memorial Sloan-Kettering Cancer Center (Yagoda 1977), lymphangiography was found to be inaccurate for repetitive assessment of tumor size. Survival time can also be an inadequate endpoint for this cancer. However, the serum carcinoembryonic antigen (CEA) level can be helpful; a value greater than 5 ng% is found in 50%–60% of cases and in over 90% of these, a falling CEA level correlates with objective tumor regression (Yagoda 1977; 1980).

The addition of cyclophosphamide to cisplatin produced responses in 43% of cases (Yagoda et al. 1978). In a variety of clinical trials which combined cisplatin and adriamycin, 30 (42%) of 72 cases responded (Yagoda 1980). In 94 adequately treated patients who received cisplatin, adriamycin and cyclophosphamide in various dosages and schedules, the overall response rate was 41%. The latter three-drug combination regimen (CISCA) was reported initially (Sternberg et al. 1977) to have induced remission in 12 (87%) of 14 patients, but as additional cases were studied, the response rate decreased to the 42%–50% range (Samuels 1979). The CISCA protocol was rather toxic and required dose modifications because of marked myelosuppression and a relatively high incidence of sepsis. Williams et al. (1979a; 1979b) examined the combination of cisplatin, adriamycin and 5-fluorouracil. In 44 adequately treated patients, 18 (41%) responded. Thus, all cisplatin combination regimens have reported responses of approximately 35%–45% — a remission rate within the 95% confidence limits of cisplatin used singly.

The average duration of remission for most combination regimens is slightly longer — 2 months, but some investigators have described a higher incidence of complete remissions (Samuels 1979). Currently, large randomized trials are evaluating cisplatin vs. cisplatin and cyclophosphamide, and cisplatin vs. cisplatin and adriamycin. Preliminary data do not indicate any significant additive or synergistic effects with such combinations. At this time, the practising oncologist should feel comfortable in using cisplatin alone. Until data are available to indicate substantial benefit with the potentially more toxic drug regimens, combination therapy should be avoided. Since patients in this age group (60–70 years) do not readily tolerate multi-drug programs, the simplest and most effective therapy should be employed.

New, as well as old drugs need to be evaluated, and in the future, new combinations (eg, cisplatin and methotrexate, cisplatin and vinblastine, etc.) might be more effective than single agents. In addition, combination drug regimens may be required based on the selective responsiveness of metastastic lesions at various sites. For example, cisplatin appears to induce more responses in nodal, subcutaneous, cutaneous, and pulmonary lesions, while methotrexate seems more effective in controlling loco-regional and intravesical disease. In these circumstances, a rationale would exist for a combination drug regimen.

Conclusion

A few agents, such as cisplatin and methotrexate, have been found consistently to induce clinically useful remissions and a 9–12 month prolongation of life for responders compared to non-responders (Yagoda 1980; Natale et al. 1981). Since cisplatin, methotrexate, adriamycin and probably mitomycin C have been shown to be effective anti-tumor agents for transitional cell carcinoma, patients with disseminated bladder cancer can now be considered for chemotherapy, where clinically appropriate.

When drugs are effective in advanced disease, hopefully the use of such agents prophylactically, in the treatment of patients with minimal disease, will produce a significant prolongation of life. At least 50%–60% of patients who are surgically staged and treated with preoperative irradiation followed by radical cystectomy die within 5 years (Cummings et al. 1979). Selected groups of patients who manifest down-staging, that is, histologically verified reduction in the extent of tumor after irradiation, have a high 5-year survival rate — in some series, 60%–70% of patients without disease (Van der Werf-Messing 1975). However, most patients show little evidence of down-staging and possibly adjuvant chemotherapy could increase survival and delay tumor recurrence. At present, randomized trials are evaluating chemotherapy vs. no chemotherapy in such groups.

Since the efficacy of adjuvant therapy is unknown and the natural history of bladder cancer remains indeterminate, stratification for good and poor risk factors is required before randomization. Patients with high grade T3 and T4, NO lesions (stages B2 and C) should benefit from intensive chemotherapy. In particular, a systemic approach is needed in patients with stages B2 and C disease who show no evidence of histological down-staging after radiation therapy or who have stage D (N1; metastases to regional lymph nodes) bladder cancer. In the latter group, the overall survival remains dismal. Of 134 patients with stage D bladder cancer treated at Memorial Sloan-Kettering Cancer Center, 50% died in 8–14 months, 7% survived 5 years, and 82% died from their disease: 38% with distant metastases alone and 25% with a pelvic recurrence only (Smith and Whitmore in press). Since the present intensive therapy aimed at control of loco-regional disease is moderately effective, further improvement in survival must rely on adjuvant chemotherapy for control of systemic micro-metastases.

References

Al-Sarraf M, Amer MH, Vaitkevicius VK (1977) Chemotherapy and survival in patients with urinary bladder cancer. Proc Am Assoc Cancer Res 18: 116

Burnard KG, Boyd PJR, Mayo ME (1976) Single-dose intravesical thiotepa as an adjuvant to cystodiathermy in the treatment of transitional cell bladder carcinoma. Br J Urol 48: 55–59

Carter SK (1978) Chemotherapy and senitorurinary oncology. Cancer Treat Rev 5: 85–93

Cohen SM (1979) Urinary bladder carcinogenesis: Initiation — promotion. Semin Oncol 6: 157–160

Cross RJ, Glashan RW, Humphrey CS, Robinson MRG, Smith PH, Williams RE (1976) Treatment of advanced bladder cancer with adriamycin and 5-fluorouracil. Br J Urol 48: 609–615

Cummings KB, Shipley WM, Einstein AB, Cutler SJ (1979) Current concepts in the management of patients with deeply invasive bladder carcinoma. Semin Oncol 6: 220–228

Duchek M, Edsymr F, Naeslund I (1980) 5-Fluorouracil in the treatment of recurrent cancer of the urinary bladder. In: Pavone-Macaluso M, Smith PH, Edsmyr F (eds) Bladder tumors and other topics in urological oncology. Plenum Press, New York, pp 381–385

Early K, Elias EG, Mittelman A, Albert D, Murphy GP (1973) Mitomycin C in the treatment of metastatic transitional cell carcinoma of the bladder. Cancer 31: 1150–1153

EORTC (1972) Clinical screening of epipodophyllotoxin VM-26 in malignant lymphomas and solid tumors. Br Med J ii: 744–748

EORTC (1977) The treatment of advanced carcinoma of the bladder with a combination of adriamycin and 5-fluorouracil. Eur Urol 3: 276–278

Farrow GM (1979) Pathologist's role in bladder cancer. Semin Oncol 6: 198–206

Gad-el-Mawla N, Chevlen E, Hamza R, Ziegler JL (1979) Phase II trial of cis-dichlorodiammineplatinum (II) in cancer of the Bilharzial bladder. Cancer Treat Rep 63: 1577–1578

Hall RR, Bloom HJG, Freeman JE, Nawrocki A, Wallace DM, (1974) Methotrexate treatment for advanced bladder cancer. Br J Urol 46: 431–438

Herr H (1980) Diamminedichloride platinum II in the treatment of advanced bladder cancer. J Urol 123: 953–955

Mechl Z, Rovny F, Sopkova B (1977) VM-26 (4-demethyleppodophyllotoxin-beta-d-thenylidine glucoside) in the treatment of urinary bladder tumors. Neoplasma 24: 411–414

Merrin CE (1979) Treatment of genitourinary tumors with cis-dichlorodiammineplatinum (II): Experience in 250 patients. Cancer Treat Rep 63: 1579–1584

Merrin C, Cartagena R, Wajsman Z, Baumgartner G, Murphy GP (1975) Chemotherapy of bladder carcinoma with cyclophosphamide and adriamycin. J. Urol 114: 884–887

Murphy WM, Soloway MS (1980) The effect of Thio-Tepa on developed and established mammalian bladder tumors. Cancer 45: 870–875

Natale RB, Yagoda A, Watson RC, Stover DE (1980) Phase II trial of neocarzinostatin in patients with bladder and prostatic cancer: Toxicity of a 5-day IV bolus schedule. Cancer 45: 2836–2842

Natale R, Yagoda A, Watson RC, Whitmore WF, Blumenreich M, Braun D Jr (1981) Methotrexate: An active agent in bladder cancer. Cancer 47: 1246–1250

Nissen NI, Pajak TF, Leone LA, Bloomfield CD, Kennedy BJ, Ellison RR, Silver RT, Weiss RB, Cuttner J, Falkson G, Kung F, Bersevin PR, Holland JF (1980) Clinical trial of VP 16-213 (NSC 14150) IV twice weekly in advanced neoplastic disease. Cancer 45: 232–235

O'Bryan RM, Baker LH, Gottlieb JE, Rivkin SE, Bascerzak SP, Grument GN, Salmon SE, Moon TE, Hoogstraten B (1977) Dose response evaluation of adriamycin in human neoplasia. Cancer 39: 1940–1948

Oliver RTD (1980) The place of chemotherapy in the treatment of patients with invasive carcinoma of the bladder. In: Pavone-Macaluso M, Smith PH, Edsmyr F (eds) Bladder tumors and other topics in urological oncology. Plenum Press, New York, pp 381–385

Pavone-Macaluso M, and EORTC Genitourinary Tract Cooperative Group A (1976) Single drug chemotherapy of bladder cancer with adriamycin. VM-26 or bleomycin. A Phase II multicentric cooperative study. Eur Urol 2: 138–141

Rodriguez LH, Johnson DE, Holoye PY, Samuels MD (1977) Combination VM-26 and adriamycin for metastatic transitional cell carcinoma. Cancer Treat Rep 61: 187–188

Sakamato S, Ogata J, Ikegami K, Naeda H (1978) Effects of systemic administration of neocarsinostatin, a new protein antibiotic on human bladder cancer. Cancer Treat rep 62: 453–454

Samuels ML (1979) CISCA combination chemotherapy. In: Johnson DE, Samuels ML (eds) Second Annual Conference on Cancer of the Genitourinary Tract. Raven Press, New York, pp 97–106

Schellhammer Pf, Whitmore WF (1976) Transitional cell carcinoma of the urethra in men having cystectomy for bladder cancer. J Urol 115: 56–60

Smith JA, Whitmore WF (to be published) Regional lymph node metastases from bladder cancer. J Urol

Soloway MS (1978) cis-Diamminedichloroplatinum (II) (DDP) in advanced bladder cancer. J Urol 120: 716–719

Soloway MS, Murphy WM (1979) Experimental chemotherapy of bladder cancer-systemic and intravesical. Semin Oncol 6: 166–183

Sternberg JJ, Bracken RB, Handel PB, Johnson DE (1977) Combination chemotherapy (Cisca) for advanced urinary tract carcinoma. A preliminary report. JAMA 238: 2282–2287

Turner AG, Hendry WF, Williams GB, Bloom HJG (1977) The treatment of advanced bladder cancer with methotrexate. Br J Urol 49: 673–678

Van der Werf Messing B (1975) Carcinoma of the bladder T-3, M-x, N-o treated by pre-operative irradiation followed by cystectomy. Cancer 36: 718–722

Whitmore WF (1979) Surgical management of low stage bladder cancer. Semin Oncol 6: 207–216

Williams SD, Donohue JP, Einhorn LH (1979a) Advanced bladder cancer: Therapy with cis-dichlorodiammine platinum (II), adriamycin and 5-fluorouracil. Cancer Treat Rep 63: 1573–1576

Williams SD, Einhorn LH, Donohue JP (1979b) cis-Platinum combination chemotherapy of bladder cancer. Cancer Clin Trials 2: 335–338

Yagoda A (1977) Future implications of phase 2 chemotherapy trials in ninety-five patients with measurable advanced bladder cancer. Cancer Res 37: 2275–2280

Yagoda A (1980) Chemotherapy of metastatic bladder cancer. Cancer 45: 1879–1888

Yagoda A, Watson RC, Gonzalez-Vitale JC, Grabstald H, Whitmore W (1976) cis-Dichlorodiammineplatinum (II) in advanced bladder cancer. Cancer Treat Rep 60: 917–923

Yagoda A, Watson RC, Grabstald H, Barzell WE, Whitmore WF (1977a) Adriamycin and cyclophosphamide in advanced bladder cancer. Cancer Treat Rep 61: 97–99

Yagoda A, Watson RC, Whitmore WF, Grabstald H, Middleman MP, Krakoff IH (1977b) Adriamycin in advanced urinary tract cancer: Experience in 42 patients and a review of the literature. Cancer 39: 279–285

Yagoda A, Watson RC, Kemey N, Barzell WE, Grabstald H, Whitmore WF (1978) Diamminedichloride platinum II and cyclophosphamide in the treatment of advanced urothelial cancer. Cancer 41: 2121–2130

Yagoda A, Watson RC, Whitmore WF (1980) Phase II trial of methotrexate in bladder cancer. Proc Am Assoc Cancer Res 21: 427

Chapter 7

Chemotherapy of Cancer of the Prostate

F. M. Torti and S. K. Carter

Introduction

Cancer of the prostate is the second leading cause of cancer deaths among American men (Enstrom and Austin 1977; Third National Cancer Survey 1974). The expected annual incidence is 42 000 new cases with 17 000 deaths. It has been estimated that 30% of cases are potentially curable when first discovered but this is open to serious question (Klein 1979). Between 1950 and 1970 the reported incidence of prostatic carcinoma rose from 17 to 21 per 100 000 population. This rise has been mainly in American nonwhites (Ernster et al. 1978) and has been attributed to improvements in medical care, screening and accuracy of diagnosis.

In a 20-year period the 5-year survival rate has increased from 30% to 59%. This is derived from a combination of increasing incidence and an age-adjusted mortality rate which has dropped from 7.5 deaths to 7.0 deaths per 100 000 population. This increased survival is due mainly to an increase in newly diagnosed 'occult' lesions which have a minimal lethal potential. When metastatic disease is present at diagnosis, the interval between diagnosis and death averages less than 3 years and has not changed with time (Nesbit and Plumb 1946; VA Cooperative Urological Research Group 1967).

Therapy has been in transition as a combination of new surgical techniques, the evaluation of radiotherapy, and the development of modestly effective chemotherapy have increased the number of options for treatment. New diagnostic methods and a greater elucidation of prostate cancer's natural history has improved the classification of this tumor, enabling more precise treatment prescriptions to be developed.

Staging, Surgery and Radiotherapy

Most patients with prostatic cancer are diagnosed because of symptoms of obstruction or symptoms from metastatic lesions (Whitmore 1963). Only about one in ten diagnoses are made examining tissue removed for apparently benign disease (Labess 1952). Whitmore (1963) reported that over 80% of his patients had advanced tumors at diagnosis.

The staging of cancer of the prostate is now becoming more precise. For over 20 years a four-stage classification has been used which was originally presented by Whitmore (1956). This has been expanded to seven stages through the development of subclassifications (Klein 1979) (Table 7.1). In the newer classification there is a reasonable correlation between advancing stage and incidence of lymph node metastases (Table 7.2). This is highly important since ultimate disease progression correlates closely with lymph node involvement (Catalona and Scott 1978).

Table 7.1.   Staging classification of prostatic cancer

1956 Classification	1978 Modification
Clinical stage	
A Tumor not clinically detectable	A1 Well-differentiated
Discovered on pathologic examination only	A2 Poorly differentiated
B Tumor limited to the prostate	B1 Tumor <1.5 cm in diameter or 1 lobe and well-differentiated
	B2 Tumor > 1.5 cm in diameter or > 1 lobe and moderately to poorly differentiated
C Extended beyond the confines of the prostate capsule	C Disease locally extensive, acid phosphatase normal or positive, moderately to poorly differentiated
D Metastatic disease	D1 Acid phosphatase normal or + with normal bone/scan survey, positive lymph nodes below the aortic bifurcation
	D2 Positive lymph nodes above the aortic bifurcation or bony and soft tissue metastases

Table 7.2.   Correlation of 1978 staging system of prostatic cancer with frequency of lymph node metastases [a]

Clinical stage	Frequency of lymph node metastases
A1	5
A2	25
B1	8–21
B2	14–45
C	40–80
D1	100
D2	100

[a] Arduino et al. 1967, Byar 1972a.

Stage A carcinoma is defined as being unsuspected clinically. These are usually discovered during examination of a specimen removed for presumed benign prostatic hypertrophy. This type of carcinoma does not possess a uniformly good prognosis: from 7% to 40% of patients show progression of disease, with early metastases and death (Heaney et al. 1977; Byar 1972a; Emmett et al. 1960; Barnes et al. 1976). This has led to attempts to substage patients into those who will and those who will not require further therapy. Histological appearance and size appear to be the best prognosticators available. Hanash et al. (1972) have reported that patients with poorly differentiated lesions have the highest incidence of death from their malignancy. Barnes et al. (1976) reported that patients with diffuse lesions involving more than one-fourth of the gland had a high incidence of metastatic disease compared with patients having more focal lesions. Heaney et al. (1977) studied 100 patients with stage A lesions followed for at least 10 years. Eight died of carcinoma; in six of these patients the lesion was diffuse, and in seven it was moderately or poorly differentiated.

Many urologists do not recommend further treatment for stage A1 carcinoma (Heaney et al. 1977). There is no evidence that estrogens or orchiectomy prolong survival for these patients with 'the pathologists' cancer' (Barnes et al. 1976; Greene and Simon 1955). In patients with stage A2 disease therapy is indicated (Barnes et al. 1976; Golimbu et al. 1978; Byar 1972b). The therapeutic options are prostatic irradiation with supervoltage equipment to total doses of 7000 to 7600 rads at the center of the prostate (Bagshaw et al. 1975), or radical excision of the prostate (Jewett 1975). Since irradiation has been shown to be highly effective in achieving local control, in the absence of metastatic disease and when the lymph nodes are not pathologically involved, it appears to be preferable for true stage A2 disease.

Stage B lesions are defined as being totally confined to the prostate gland. This subset accounts for roughly 10% of newly discovered cases (Jewett et al. 1972). Unfortunately digital rectal examination leads to an underestimation of the extent of spread in 25%–45% of patients thought to have stage B disease (Byar and Mostofi 1972; Whitmore and MacKenzie 1959). Serum acid phosphatase will be elevated in only 5% rising to 24% in patients with ultimately proven metastases to bone (Woodward 1952; Yam 1974). Bone marrow acid phosphatase has not lived up to its early promise (Chua et al. 1970; Pontes et al. 1978; Fossa et al. 1978). Since lymph node metastases usually precede clinically evident bone metastases, skeletal X-ray surveys will grossly underestimate the problem (Rubin 1969). Radionuclide bone scans are more readily performed, less costly than skeletal radiography and are 20%–25% more sensitive in the detection of early bone disease.

It is hoped that a separation into B1 and B2 will delineate those patients who could truly be expected to be cured by effective local therapy (B1) from those likely to have microscopic bone disease presaged by lymph node involvement (Klein 1979). Again it is hoped that histology will be helpful. In the study of Barzell et al. (1977) 100 consecutive patients with clinical stage B and C lesions underwent pelvic lymph-adenectomy. Lymph node spread was observed in 16% of well-differentiated tumors, 39% of moderately well-differentiated tumors and 60% of those poorly differentiated. Tumor size may also be helpful with B1 being defined as a lesion involving less than one lobe or not greater than 1.5 cm and B2 being involvement of more than one lobe or larger than 1.5 cm in diameter.

Lymphography when carried out with care and expertly interpreted is helpful in determining the presence and extent of lymph node involvement. At Stanford an 88% correlation was initially reported (Castellino et al. 1973), but with staging lymph-adenectomy in a larger series, this correlation has fallen to 79% (Bagshaw et al. 1975). Lymphography can add important data on the extent of disease to the classical staging approach of physical examination, serum acid phosphatase estimation and radiologic bone examination. It is unresolved whether pelvic lymphadenectomy is warranted as a pathologic staging procedure. It has not been shown that lymphadenectomy is of therapeutic benefit; lymph node disease usually means subsequent metastatic dissemination. If an effective adjuvant systemic therapy is devised, the procedure might define the patient subsets who would benefit.

The therapeutic options for stage B are radical prostatectomy or external beam radiation. Both are effective for local control but have little impact on survival for those patients with nodal involvement (stage B2). Schroeder and Belt (1975) reported that radical prostatectomy for true stage B lesions results in a 15-year relapse-free survival that does not differ substantially from the expected survival of the population at large. While no data are available on untreated stage B patients Hanash et al. (1972) reported a 19% 5-year survival with transurethral resection only.

At Stanford 22% of 31 patients with clinical stage B relapsed within a 10-year follow-up after irradiation (Bagshaw et al. 1975). In a second study from Stanford (Bagshaw et al. 1977) 87% of patients without nodal metastases after lymph-adenectomy are free of overt disease with a median follow-up time of 22 months. Both irradiation and radical prostatectomy cause impotence and urinary incontin-ence although the incidence appears higher with the latter (Whitmore 1963; Jewett 1975). Radiation enteritis may be more frequent when irradiation follows surgery (Bagshaw et al. 1977).

Stage C carcinoma is defined as a lesion which on digital rectal examination has extended beyond the confines of the prostate capsule, usually into the seminal vesicles, their fascia or more distant sites. The acid phosphatase and radiologic bone surveys will be negative. These lesions account for 40% of newly diagnosed cases (Flocks et al. 1975). Nodal involvement can be pathologically documented in 63%–79% of cases with none of these surviving 5 years (Whitmore and MacKenzie 1959). Whitmore (1956) reported that 22% of stage C patients will survive 3 years without therapy. This is consistent with the reports that 21%–37% of stage C patients will have negative nodes. Local therapy alone will not be curative if regional lymph nodes are involved (Barzell et al. 1977; McCullough and Leadbetter 1972). What is needed for effective therapy is reliable clinical staging of the regional nodes and pathological staging.

Local control in stage C disease can usually be obtained with irradiation. Studies from Stanford (Ray et al. 1973) and other institutions (Hill et al. 1974) indicate local control can be achieved in 85%–90% of patients. Surgical approaches have to be extensive and appear to have higher morbidity with comparable local control in comparison to irradiation.

Stage D carcinoma includes all tumors, regardless of size or histologic pattern, that have spread beyond the prostate gland to lymph nodes, bone or viscera. Barzell et al. (1977) reported that 50% of new cases were stage D. Three therapeutic possibilities exist for these patients: watchful waiting, immediate hormonal manipulation and cytotoxic chemotherapy. Observation only is based on the belief that palliative hormonal therapy should be reserved for symptomatic patients. In symptomatic cases (outflow obstruction or severe bone pain) immediate hormonal manipulation usually is indicated, although radiation can be used in certain settings.

Hormone Manipulations

Endocrine therapy for prostatic carcinoma is among the oldest approaches to cancer treatment with systemic therapy in the modern era. Endocrine therapy has for a long time consisted of either castration or estrogen therapy. The most widely quoted series is that of the Veterans Administration Cooperative Urologic Research Group (VACURG) (Arduino et al. 1967; Arduino et al. 1978; Byar 1973) in studies of more than 2000 cases. Stage III and IV patients were randomized to placebo, 5 mg of diethylsibestrol daily, orchiectomy, or the combination of 5 mg stilbestrol daily plus orchiectomy. In stage III disease patients treated with castration and estrogens had a lower survival than the placebo group. In stage IV disease mortality was comparable in all groups. Detailed analysis of the data revealed that the estrogen treated group had a higher rate of complications and mortality due to cardiovascular disease. This more than outweighed a lowering of mortality due to cancer in the additive hormone group. When 491 patients of similar age and cardiovascular status were compared, 24% of those receiving placebo compared to 39% of the stilbestrol treated patients developed severe or fatal cardiovascular complications, mainly myocardial infarctions and cerebrovascular accidents. Forty percent of the estrogen treated men developed these complications within 1 year of starting therapy.

A follow-up study by the VACURG compared various lower doses of stilbestrol (0.2 mg and 1.0 mg daily) with 5.0 mg and placebo. They found that 1.0 mg daily was as effective as 5 mg daily in delaying progression, and that the lower dose was associated with fewer cardiovascular deaths. In patients with advanced disease both 1.0 and 5.0 mg were more effective in tumor control than 0.2 mg or placebo. Mackler et al. (1972) have observed that 1 mg is as effective as 5 mg in lowering plasma testosterone, but Shearer et al. (1973) and Kent et al. (1973) indicated that testosterone suppression with the 1 mg daily dose was variable.

Chemotherapy

Criteria of Response

Any review of prostatic carcinoma chemotherapy is made difficult by the problem of response criteria and the lack of comparable criteria among various groups studying the disease. In prostatic cancer most patients do not have a tumor mass encompassable by calipers. It is therefore necessary to define response with less precise measurements. These have included stabilization of disease, subjective improvement, and changes in acid phosphatase. The VACURG attempted to avoid the problem by using survival as their major end point. Even where measurable disease is present there exists no standard definition of partial response (Table 7.3). Stabilization as a response measurement is open to potential observer bias in its scoring and possibly lacks biological significance.

That stabilization may be a meaningful end point is supported by data from the NPCP that patients who are stable survive almost as long as patients who have clear cut objective regressions. In addition the duration of response is comparable in both groups.

The major problem in data comparison is the incorporation of stabilization with partial response in overall reported response rates. The NPCP (Scott et al. 1967) defines a responder as a patient who shows a partial regression or stabilization of disease. Their overall response rate often combines these two criteria. An example of the problem can be seen in their data with estramustine. They report a 30% response rate with only 3 of 46 patients (7%) achieving a partial regression of tumor (Murphy et al. 1977). Which of these two response rates is the more biologically significant is uncertain.

Not only the inclusion of stabilization in response rate, but also the definition of partial response, makes data comparison difficult. The NPCP has a rigorous definition of partial response requiring both 50% reduction of tumor size and normalization of acid phosphatase (Scott et al. 1967; Murphy et al. 1977; Scott et al. 1975; Scott et al. 1976; Schmidt et al. 1976; Schmidt et al. 1979). With these criteria, objective reponse with cyclophosphamide was observed in only 3 of 41 cases. If only a 50% reduction in primary tumor size is required, the response rate would be 31%, comparable with that reported in other studies with cyclophosphamide.

Table 7.3. Partial response criteria

Response sites	Study groups					
	Uro-Oncology Group	NPCP	ECOG	SWOG	NCI-VA	NCOG
Tumor						
50% Measurable area	X	X	X	X	X	X
Acid phosphatase						
Return to normal	X	X				
50% Reduction			X	X	X	X
Alkaline phosphatase						
Return to normal	X	X				
50% Reduction			X	X	NS	X
Functional status						
Weight must not significantly decrease	X	X	NS	X	X	X
Performance status must not decrease	X	X	NS	X	X	X
Bones						
Recalcification of lytic bone lesions	X	X	NS	NS	NS	NS
Concomitant radiation for pain	NS	NS	no	yes	NS	yes

NS: Not specified or unknown.

The interpretation of acid phosphatase levels still remains controversial. As a tumor marker acid phosphatase is of limited value; it is elevated in 60%–75% of patients with documented bony metastases (Schaffer and Pendergrass 1976; Johnson et al. 1976). On the other hand sequential study during treatment does appear to have some prognostic value. There have been attempts to correlate initial elevation with survival. In some series the higher the initial level the shorter the survival, but this has not been a universal finding (Johnson et al. 1976; Byar 1977; Ishihe et al. 1974). Failure of elevated values to diminish after treatment with hormones or drugs usually correlates with short survival.

The correlation between measurable tumor shrinkage and diminished acid phosphatase also is not clearly established. In the studies of the NPCP they did correlate with each other (Johnson et al. 1976). On the other hand in the studies of the Eastern Cooperative Oncology Group they did not, although both independently predicted for survival (deWys and Begg 1978). The biological meaning of an increased acid phosphatase is not fully established. It may be related to tumor mass, to tumor differentiation, or to other factors.

Difficulties in Interpretation of Results

Several prognostic variables have been elucidated as potentially important in advanced prostatic cancer under treatment. The VACURG has emphasized the importance of histologic grade (Gleason and Mellinger 1974; Gleason 1977). In addition they found that poor survival correlated with advanced clinical stage, ureteric obstruction, anemia and progression to, as opposed to diagnosis with, stage IV disease (Housepian and Byar 1976; Arduino et al. 1968). The NPCP (Schmidt et al. 1976) has added bone marrow biopsy evidence of tumor, prior radiation therapy and abnormal liver-spleen scan to the list of poor prognostic indicators. In the ECOG studies performance status was important as was anemia and prior radiation (DeWys et al. 1977).

Another problem in the interpretation of prostatic cancer treatment data is the impact of death from intercurrent illness. In the studies of the VACURG, death from other conditions occurred in 40% of stage III patients and 35% of stage IV patients. These deaths can easily obscure treatment differences when overall survival is used as an end point.

Large numbers of patients are required to demonstrate significant differences between treatment groups: this is partly because of the number of patients with clinically insignificant prostatic cancer, who will either die with microscopic, but not clinical disease, or whose clinically apparent disease is so indolent it will not adversely affect survival (Byar 1972a). Unfortunately these patients are not easily separated out before beginning therapy. The most potent indicators appear to be low clinical stage and low histologic grade.

Single Agent Chemotherapy

Cyclophosphamide is one of the most studied drugs. The total cumulative response rate in 125 patients was 32% (Table 7.4). This includes 34 patients treated before 1973 in studies not specifically designed for prostatic cancer. The rest of the data comes predominantly from the National Prostatic Cancer Project (NPCP) studies (Scott et al. 1967; Scott et al. 1975; Scott et al. 1976; Schmidt et al. 1976; Schmidt et al. 1979). In their first study they compared cyclophosphamide to 5-fluorouracil (5-FU) and 'standard' therapy in patients who had not received irradiation. Standard therapy was defined as any non-cytotoxic treatment such as prednisone, radiation or chlorotrianisene. A cross-over design was used at 12 weeks between the two chemotherapy regimens. Most of the patients had been treated with orchiectomy (70%). In this study cyclophosphamide gave a 46% response rate in 41 patients utilizing criteria which include stabilization in the overall response calculation. In a later study cyclophosphamide was compated to dicarbazine (DTIC) and pro-carbazine. In this study the response rate fell to 26% in 35 cases. A difference was also observed in pain relief between the two studies. In the first study pain relief occurred in 54% of the patients treated with cyclophosphamide; in the second study it was only 23%. The Western Cancer Study Group (Chlebowsky et al. 1979), using criteria similar to that of the NPCP (including stabilization) reported a 53% response rate for cyclophosphamide.

Table 7.4.   Cyclophosphamide in prostatic cancer.

Group	No. of patients	No. resp.	% Response	References
NPCP				
Protocol 100	41	18[a]	46	[b]
Protocol 300	35	9[a]	26	[c]
Western Group	15	8[a]	53	[d]
Cumulative data prior to 1973	34	4	12	[e]
Total	125	40	32	

[a] Response includes stabilization.
[b] Ishiha et al. 1974; Jewett 1975; Jewett et al. 1972; Johnson et al. 1976.
[c] Jonsson and Hogberg 1971.
[d] Merrin 1978a.
[e] Merrin 1978b.

Table 7.5. 5-Fluorouracil in prostatic cancer

Group	No. of patients	No. resp.	% resp.	References
NPCP Protocol 100	33	12[a]	36	[b]
ECOG	40	3	8	[c]
NCI-VA	8	2	25	[d]
Cumulative data prior to 1973	39	10	27	[e]
Total	120	27	23	

[a] Response includes stabilization.
[b] Ishihe et al. 1974; Jewett 1975; Jewett et al. 1972; Johnson et al. 1976.
[c] Klein 1979.
[d] Mittelman et al. 1976; Muntzing et al. 1974.
[e] Merrin 1962.

5-FU has a cumulative response rate of 23% in a total of 120 patients (Table 7.5). This includes 39 patients (with ten responses) in earlier (pre-1973) studies where response criteria were poorly defined and prognostic variables as related to prostate cancer unavailable. The NPCP (Scott et al. 1967; Scott et al. 1975; Scott et al. 1976; Schmidt et al. 1976) observed a 36% response rate in 33 patients. The ECOG (DeWys and Begg 1978; DeWys 1975; DeWys et al. 1977) saw only an 8% response rate in 40 patients while the NCI-VA Group (Tejada et al. 1977a,b) reported two responses in eight patients. If the response rate to 5-FU focuses only on the post-1973 era, and studies which excluded stabilization in the response criteria, then the response rate is only 10% (5/48).

When objective response rate is examined, excluding stabilization, then adriamycin appears to be one of the most active single agents (Table 7.6). In the study of the ECOG (DeWys and Begg 1978; DeWys 1975; DeWys et al. 1977) adriamycin gave a 24% response rate in 38 patients. In the ECOG study 16% of the adriamycin-treated group had a 50% decrease in acid phosphatase. The median survival was 31 weeks in comparison to 23 weeks in a group of patients treated with 5-FU. As indicated earlier, the 5-FU study has a very low response rate yet overall the two groups had a similar (not statistically different) survival.

In the phase II evaluation of adriamycin by the Southwest Oncology Group (O'Bryan et al. 1977), the response rate in prostatic cancer in good risk patients was 3/10 at 75 mg/m^2, 2/4 at 60 mg/m^2 and 0/5 at 45 mg/m^2. The overall response rate for the good risk groups was 5/19 (26%) and if one excludes the low dose this increases to

Table 7.6. Adriamycin in prostatic cancer

Group	No. eval. patients	No. resp.	% resp.	References
Southwest Oncology Group				[a]
Good risk	19	5	26	
Poor risk	19	0	0	
Eastern Cooperative Oncology Group	38	9	24	[b]
Mayo Clinic	19	5	26	[c]
Total	95	19	20	

[a] Murphy et al. 1977.
[b] Klein 1979; Merrin and Beckley 1979; Mittelman et al. 1975.
[c] Nagel and Kollin 1976, 1977.

34% (5/14). There were no responses in the poor risk group treated at either 50 mg/m^2 (7 patients) or 25 mg/m^2 (12 patients). At the Mayo Clinic (Egan et al. 1975; Egan et al. 1976) adriamycin gave a 19% response rate in 26 patients. Thus the overall response rate is 20% (19/95) (Table 7.6). If one excludes the poor risk and low dose patients of the Southwest Oncology Group then the response rate increases to 27% (17/71).

Among other classes of drugs the nitrosoureas have undergone some study. BCNU has a response rate of 1/8 from older studies while CCNU gave responses in 4/10 in the NCI-VA study (Tejada et al. 1977a,b). Streptozotocin in the NPCP study (Murphy et al. 1977) gave a response rate of 32% in 38 patients yet none of these patients had objective tumor shrinkage.

Cisplatin (cis-platinum diamminedichloride II) has been studied at Roswell Park (Merrin 1978b; Merrin and Beckley 1979) with 29% responding out of 45 treated. Another six patients had stable disease and 40% had appreciable reduction in bone pain.

One of the more interesting new drugs is estramustine, in which nitrogen mustard is linked to estradiol (Jönsson and Hogberg 1971; Alfthan and Rusk 1969). In animals it has been shown that the estrogen moiety serves as a carrier for the alkylator. A specific cytotoxic effect is presumed to occur when the estrogen moiety is sequestered in cells with estrogen receptors (Kadohama et al. 1978; Muntzing et al. 1974). There is indirect evidence that estrogenic effects occur as well (Fossa and Miller 1976; VonHoff et al. 1977). Gynecomastia is observed in patients treated with estramustine, even in those without prior hormonal manipulation. Elevated plasma levels of estrogens have been demonstrated in patients on the drug, as well as concomitant decrease in plasma testosterone levels (Fossa and Miller 1976). Changes in luteinizing hormone and follicle stimulating hormone have also been described (Edsmyr et al. 1978).

Estramustine was originally introduced into clinical study in Sweden (Anderson 1975; Nagel and Kollin 1976, 1977; Lindberg 1972; Nilsson and Jonsson 1975), and has also been studied in the U.S. and Britain (Mittelman et al. 1975, 1976; Chisholm et al. 1977; Merrin et al. 1976; Merrin 1978a). The drug has been used in patients who failed on conventional hormone therapy and also in selected patients as primary treatment for stage D disease. It can be given by either intravenous or oral routes. Several studies have reported responses in about half the patients treated. The duration of response has ranged from 3 to 36 months. Intravenous administration has caused severe local phlebitis. Although some studies suggest a higher response rate by the IV route, confirmation is necessary, especially given the local toxicity of this route. In patients without previous hormone therapy response rates of 63% and 83% have been reported. The critical question that remains unanswered is how would this compare with estrogen alone?

The NPCP compared estramustine to streptozotocin in patients with extensive irradiation. A third arm of 'standard' therapy was given as discussed earlier. The overall response rate with estramustine was 33% but if only objective shrinkage is looked at this falls to 3/46 (7%), compared to 32% overall for streptozotocin with no objective shrinkage observed. The duration of response was significantly longer for estramustine (45 weeks) as compared to streptozotocin (31 weeks) and 'standard' therapy (30 weeks).

Prednimustine, an ester of chlorambucil and prednisone has also been tested in hormone-resistant prostatic cancer. Catane et al. (1977, 1978) reported objective regressions in 3 of 23 patients (13%) with 8 showing subjective improvement. The same group has also combined prednimustine with estramustine but the response rate does not appear to be higher.

A summary of available single agent data from trials since 1973 designed specifically for prostatic cancer is given in Table 7.7. The data are broken down by whether stabilization is included in the overall response rate (group A) or is excluded (group B). Among agents not previously mentioned are procarbazine with a 14% response rate in an NPCP evaluation (Schmidt et al. 1979) and DTIC with a 39% response rate. Melphalan, in a study of the Yorkshire urologic group (Houghton et al. 1977), produced only one objective regression among 15 evaluable patients. The only agent with more than 100 cases is estramustine which has been extensively studied in Europe.

Table 7.7. Overall response rate for single agents in prostatic cancer

	Group A[a]			Group B[b]		
	No. patients	No. responses	% responses	No. patients	No. responses	% responses
5-Fluorouracil	33	12	36	48	5	10
Cyclophosphamide	76	28	37			
Adriamycin				83	19	23
Cis-platinum				45	12	29
DTIC	23	9	39			
Procarbazine	21	3	14			
CCNU				10	4	40
Melphalan				15	1	7
Streptozotocin	38	12	32			
Estramustine	30	8	29	319	56	18
Prednimustine				23	3	13

[a] Group A: Response rate for studies which include the NPCP 'stabilization' in overall response rate.
[b] Group B: Studies which exclude 'stabilization' from response rate.

Table 7.8 looks at the modern single agent data broken down by the individual studies. The most extensive data comes from the NPCP. Their protocol 100 demonstrates a convincing value for cytotoxic drugs. Not only did drugs give some objective tumor regression but the number of patients who continued with progressive disease in spite of therapy was fewer in the chemotherapy than in the standard treatment groups. The chemotherapy group also had better pain relief. Pain relief was recorded in only 26% of the patients in the standard or hormonal treatment group; in the chemotherapy group it occurred in 60% of patients.

When survival was analyzed it was demonstrated that responders lived longer than non-responders, the median for the former being 60–80 weeks as compared to 40 weeks for the non-responder. This tendency to longer survival was reflected not only in the responding patients but also in those with stable disease.

The available early chemotherapy data from general solid tumor studies are given in Table 7.9. Much of this data was published before 1970 and the response criteria are poorly defined. There is evidence for alkylating agent activity which has been confirmed. The report of activity for intralesional triethylene thiophosphoramide in refractory local disease has not been confirmed.

Combination Chemotherapy

Several combinations of chemotherapeutic agents have been tried, the most effective appearing to be combinations including either adriamycin or cyclophosphamide

Table 7.8. Single agents tabulated by study group (Studies post 1973)

Investigator	Drug	No. patients evaluable	Reported objective response rate (%)	References
NPCP 100	5-FU	33	36%[a]	[b]
	Cyclophosphamide	41	46[a]	
	Standard hormonal	36	19[a]	
NPCP 200	Estramustine	46	33[a]	[c]
	Streptozotocin	38	32[a]	
	Standard hormonal	31	19[a]	
NPCP 300	DTIC	55	27[a]	[d]
	Procarbazine	39	14[a]	
	Cyclophosphamide	35	26[a]	
ECOG	Adriamycin	38	24	[e]
	5-FU	40	8	
NCI-VA	5-FU	8	25	[f]
	CCNU	10	40	
Roswell Park	cis-Platinum	45	29	[g]
Yorkshire Urologic Group	Melphalan	15	7	[h]
Roswell Park	Prednimustine	23	13[a]	[i]
SWOG Phase II	Adriamycin			[j]
	Good risk	19	26	
	Poor risk	19	0	

[a] Used NPCP Response Criteria which include stabilization in overall response.
[b] Ishihe et al. 1964; Jewett 1975; Jewett et al. 1972; Johnson et al. 1976.
[c] Izbecki et al. 1978.
[d] Jonson and Hogberg 1971.
[e] Klein 1979; Merrin and Beckley 1979; Mittelman et al. 1975.
[f] Mittelman et al. 1976; Muntzing et al. 1974.
[g] Nesbit and Plumb 1946; Nilsson and Johnsson 1975.
[h] VACURG 1967; Vonttoff et al. 1977.
[i] Third National Cancer Survey 1974; Van Amburg et al. 1979.
[j] Murphy et al. 1977.

Table 7.9. Chemotherapeutic agents[a] before 1973

	No. treated	No. of responses
Alanine mustard	29	4
BCNU	8	1
Cyclophosphamide	34	4
5-Fluorouracil	39	10
Methotrexate	24	3
Mithramycin	21	1
Vincristine	12	1
Fluorodeoxyuridine	8	3

[a] Only agents studied in more than seven adequately treated patients.

(Table 7.10). Although response rates are somewhat higher than with single agents, evidence of superiority to single agents in controlled trials is lacking.

The Mayo Clinic group has employed adriamycin alone for a reported objective response rate of 26% in 19 patients, while the combination of cyclophosphamide and 5-fluorouracil provided a response rate of 11% in 18 patients (Eagan et al. 1975,

Table 7.10. Combination therapy and combination therapy vs single agents

Drug	No. patients evaluable	Reported objective response rate (%)[e]	Investigator	References
Adriamycin	19	26	Mayo Clinic	[b]
Cyclophosphamide + 5-FU	18	11		
Hydroxyurea + TACE	30	50[a]	Lerner	[c]
Adriamycin + cyclophosphamide	20	69[a]	Roswell Park	[d]
5-FU + cyclophosphamide	13	65[a]		
5-FU + MTX + vincristine + melphalan + prednisone	25	24	Duke	[e]
Adriamycin + cis-platinum	17	53	Mt. Sinai– Dartmouth– U. of Minn.	[f]
Adriamycin + cyclophosphamide	15	69[a]	Wayne State	[g]
Adriamycin + cyclophosphamide	18	33	NCI-VA	[h]
Estramustine + 5-FU	25	32	Yale	[i]
Cyclophosphamide vs	15	53[a]	Western Cancer Study Group	[j]
Cyclophosphamide + adriamycin + 5-FU	12	50[a]		
Adriamycin + BCNU + cyclophosphamide	22	32	Washington U., (St. Louis)	[k]
Estramustine + prednimustine	21	24	Roswell Park	[l]

[a] Used NPCP Response Criteria which include stabilization in overall response.
[b] Eagan et al. 1975, 1976.
[c] Lerner and Malloy 1977.
[d] Merrin et al. 1976.
[e] Paulson et al. 1978.
[f] Perloff et al. 1977.
[g] Izbecki et al. 1978.
[h] Idhe et al. 1978.
[i] Kennealey et al. 1978.
[j] Chlebowsky et al. 1979.
[k] Van Amburg et al. 1979.
[l] Byar 1972b.

1976). The Roswell Park group, using objective response rates which include stable disease, obtained rates of 69% and 65% for combinations of adriamycin plus cyclophosphamide and 5-fluorouracil plus cyclophosphamide, respectively (Merrin et al. 1976). This study was not randomized. The duration of response was approximately 8 months in both groups. The Western Cancer Study Group was unable to show superiority of cyclophosphamide plus adriamycin plus 5-fluorouracil over cyclophosphamide alone. Median survival of both groups was approximately 8 months. Among the cyclophosphamide responders, median survival was 18.6 months compared to 8.1 months for those responding to combination therapy ($P < 0.05$) (Chlebowsky et al. 1979).

Two groups have studied adriamycin and cyclophosphamide. Wayne State reported a 69% response rate (Izbecki et al. 1978), and the NCI-VA group a 33% response rate (Ihde et al. 1978). Pain relief occurred in 33% of patients in the former series, and in 70%–80% of the latter group. At least part of this difference in objective response is explained by difference in response definition; the Wayne State group included 'stabilization' in their reported responses.

Other responses to combination chemotherapy include a 32% response rate to adriamycin, cyclophosphamide and BCNU (VanAmburg et al. 1979), 32% to estramustine plus 5-fluorouracil (Kennealey et al. 1978), 24% to estramustine plus prednimustine (Catane et al. 1977) and 24% for a five-drug regimen of 5-fluoro-uracil, methotrexate, vincristine, melphalan and prednisone (Paulson et al. 1978; Kane et al. 1977).

Excluding stable responses the highest reported response rate has been to the combination of adriamycin and cis-platinum (53%), although the numbers are small and follow-up brief (Perloff et al. 1977).

Conclusions

When compared to other solid tumors, the quantity and quality of data available on the chemotherapy of prostatic cancer are limited. Conclusions must therefore be tentative. Six chemotherapeutic agents stand out among those tested. Cyclo-phosphamide has had the most extensive trials. It is superior to secondary hormonal maneuvers once orchiectomy or estrogens have failed, and slightly more efficacious than 5-fluorouracil, to which it was compared in an NPCP protocol. Adriamycin has also been studied extensively and appears to have an objective response rate of about 25%. CCNU and DTIC have not been as thoroughly evaluated, but appear promising. Estramustine has been somewhat disappointing in the United States trials, but has been used in patients with extensive prior radiation, a poor prognostic group. Its toxicity is manageable and distinct from that of most other chemo-therapeutic agents. Cis-platinum may be the most active single agent in prostatic cancer if the early, dramatic results are confirmed by other investigators. Several studies are in progress. These are listed in Table 7.11.

There is no definitive evidence of superiority of combination chemotherapy over single agents; some studies suggest increased benefit, others show no advantage. Agents have not always been used in optimal dosage in combinations. Nonetheless, as more toxic combinations evolve, adequate comparison to single agents will be critical if the maximum therapeutic index is to be achieved.

A critical attitude remains essential in assessing the reported results of chemo-therapy in cancer of the prostate. Some impressive response rates are from series in which stabilization of disease was scored as a response. The value to the patient of such stabilization is questionable unless it is associated with improved quality or length of survival, and both these effects are difficult to evaluate with accuracy. The general urologist who contemplates chemotherapy for specific patients with cancer of the prostate should if possible enter the patients into an organized study and thereby contribute to the compilation of more reliable data for future guidance in this disease.

Trials of chemotherapy have concentrated upon patients with end stage prostatic cancer, many of whom have received both hormonal therapy and radiation. These trials have served to identify agents with modest or promising activity, but provide no information on the possible role of chemotherapy *early* in the course of the disease. There is natural reluctance to administer potentially toxic therapy to patients without overt disease, or even to asymptomatic patients with demonstrable disease, but this problem must be addressed, just as it has been in breast cancer. Adjuvant chemotherapy after apparent surgical cure, and chemotherapy for presymptomatic metastatic disease, should both be studied, but only in the setting of prospective, randomized, controlled clinical trials.

Table 7.11. Trials in progress in prostatic cancer

	Study group
Hormone failures	
Prednimustine	NPCP
Prednimustine + estramustine	
Cyclophosphamide	NPCP
MethylCCNU	
Hydroxyurea	
Hydroxyurea	SWOG
Adriamycin + cyclophosphamide	
Adriamycin	NCOG
Adriamycin + *cis*-platinum	
5-Fluorouracil	SEG
5-FU + cyclophosphamide + adriamycin	
Tamoxifen	SEG
Stable metastatic disease, hormone treated	
DES	NPCP
DES + estramustine	
DES + cyclophosphamide	
First treatment of metastatic disease	
DES/orchiectomy	NPCP
DES + cyclophosphamide	
Estramustine + cyclophosphamide	
DES	NCOG
DES + adriamycin	
DES	SEG
DES + cyclophosphamide	
Adjuvant therapy	
No treatment	NPCP
Cyclophosphamide	
Estramustine	

References

Alfthan OS, Rusk J (1969) Estracyt in advanced prostatic carcinoma. Ann Chir Gynaecol 58: 234–240

Anderson L (1975) International Symposium on Tumours of the Male Genital Tract, Duesseldorf, vol VII pp 24–25

Arduino L, Bailar JL, Becker L, et al. (1967) Treatment and survival of patients with cancer of the prostate. Surg Gynecol Obstet 124: 1011–1017

Arduino L, Bailar JL, Becker L, et al. (1968) Factors in the prognosis of carcinoma of the prostate: A cooperative study. J Urol 100: 59–65

Arduino L, Bailar JL, Becker L, et al. (1978) Carcinoma of the prostate — treatment comparison. J Urol 98: 516–522

Bagshaw MA, Ray GR, Pistenma DA, et al. (1975) External beam radiation therapy of primary carcinoma of the prostate. Cancer 36: 723–728

Bagshaw MA, Pistenma DA, Ray GR, et al. (1977) Evaluation of extended radiotherapy for prostatic neoplasm: 1976 progress report. Cancer Treat Rep 61: 297–306

Barnes R, Hirst A, Rosenquist R (1976) Early carcinoma of the prostate: Comparison of stages A and B. J Urol 115: 404–484

Barzell W, Bean MA, Hilaris BS, et al. (1977) Prostatic adenocarcinoma: Relationship of grade and local extent to the patterns of metastases. J Urol 118: 278–282

Byar DP (1972a) Survival of patients with incidentally found microscopic cancer of the prostate: Results of a clinical trial of conservation treatment. J Urol 108: 903–913

Byar DP (1972b) Treatment of prostatic cancer: Studies by the Veterans Administration Cooperative Urological Research Group (VACURG). Bull NY Acad Med 48: 751–766

Byar DP (1973) The Veterans Administration Cooperative Urologic Research Group studies on cancer of the prostate. Cancer 32: 1126–1130

Byar DP (1977) VACURG studies in prostatic carcinoma in urologic pathology. In: Tannenbaum M (ed) The prostate. Lea & Febiger, Philadelphia, p 241

Byar DP, Mostofi FK (1972) Carcinoma of the prostate: Prognostic evaluation of certain pathologic features in 208 radical prostatectomies (examined by the step-section technique). VACURG. Cancer 30: 5–13

Castellino RA, Ray GR, Blank N, et al. (1973) Lymphangiography in prostatic carcinoma: Preliminary observations. JAMA 223: 877–881

Catalona WJ, Scott WW (1978) Carcinoma of the prostate: A review, J Urol 119: 1–8

Catane R, Kaufman J, Mittelman A, et al. (1977) Combined therapy of advanced prostatic carcinoma with estramustine and prednimustine. J Urol 117: 332

Catane R, Kaufman JH, Madajewicz S (1978) Prednimustine therapy for advanced prostatic carcinoma. Br J Urol 50: 29–32

Chisholm GD, O'Donoghue EPN, Kennedy CL (1977) The treatment of oestrogen — escaped carcinoma of the prostate with estramustine phosphate. Br J Urol 49: 717–720

Chlebowsky RT, Hestorff R, Sadoff L, et al. (1979) Cyclophosphamide versus the combination of adriamycin, 5-fluorouracil and cyclophosphamide in the treatment of metastatic prostatic cancer. Cancer 42: 2546–2552

Chua DT, Veenema RJ, Muggia F, et al. (1970) Acid phosphatase levels in bone marrow: Value in detecting early bone metastasis from carcinoma of the prostate. J Urol 103: 462–466

DeWys WD (1975) Comparison of adriamycin (NSC-123127) and 5-fluorouracil (NSC-019893) in advanced prostatic cancer. Cancer Chemother Rep 59: 215–217

DeWys WD, Begg CB (1978) Comparison of adriamycin and 5-fluorouracil in advanced prostate cancer. Proc Am Assoc Cancer Res 19: 331

DeWys WD, Bauer M, Colsky J, Cooper RA, Creech R, Carbone PP (1977) Comparative trial of adriamycin and 5-fluorouracil in advanced prostatic cancer — Progress report. Cancer Treat Rep 61: 325–329

Eagan R, Hahn R, Myers R (1975) Adriamycin (NSC-123127) versus 5-fluorouracil (NSC-019893) and cyclophosphamide (NSC-026271) in advanced prostatic cancer: A preliminary report. Cancer Chemother Rep 59: 205–207

Eagan R, Hahn R, Myers R (1976) Adriamycin (NSC-123127) versus 5-fluorouracil (NSC-019893) and cyclophosphamide (NSC-026271) in the treatment of metastatic prostate cancer. Cancer Treat Rep 60: 115–117

Edsmyr F, Esport PL, Johansson V, et al. (1978) Clinical experimental randomized study of 2,6-cis-diphenylhexamethylcyclotetrasiloxane and estramustine-17-phosphate in the treatment of prostatic carcinoma. J Urol 120: 705–707

Emmett JL, Greene LF, Papantoniou A (1960) Endocrine therapy in carcinoma of the prostate gland: 10-year survival studies. J Urol 83: 471–484

Endostrom JE, Austin DF (1977) Interpreting cancer survival rates. Science 195: 847–857

Ernster VL, Selvin S, Winkelstein WJ Jr (1978) Cohort mortality for prostatic cancer among United States nonwhites. Science 200: 1165–1166

Flocks RH, O'Donoghue EPN, Milleman LA, et al. (1975) Management of stage C prostatic carcinoma. Urol Clin North Am 2: 163–179

Fossa SD, Miller A (1976) Treatment of advanced carcinoma of the prostate with estramustine phosphate. J Urol 115: 406–408

Fossa SD, Sokolowski J, Theodorsen L (1978) The significance of bone marrow acid phosphatase in patients with prostatic carcinoma. Br J Urol 50: 185–189

Gleason DF (1977) Histologic grading clinical staging of prostatic carcinoma in urologic pathology. In: Tannenbaum M (ed) The prostate. Lea & Febiger, Philadelphia, p 17

Gleason DF, Mellinger GT (1974) Prediction of prognosis for prostatic adenocarcinoma by combined histological grading and clinical staging. J Urol 111: 58–64

Golimbu M, Schinella R, Morales P, et al. (1978) Differences in pathological characteristics and prognosis of clinical A2 prostatic cancer from A1 and B disease. J Urol 119: 618–622

Greene LF, Simon HB (1955) Occult carcinoma of the prostate: Clinical and therapeutic study of eighty-three cases. JAMA 158: 1494–1498

Hanash KA, Utz DC, Cook EN, et al. (1972) Carcinoma of the prostate: A 15-year follow-up. J Urol 107: 450–453

Heaney JA, Change HC, Daly JJ, et al. (1977) Prognosis of clinically undiagnosed prostatic carcinoma and the influence of endocrine therapy. J Urol 118: 283–287

Hill DR, Crews QE Jr, Walsh PC (1974) Prostate carcinoma: Radiation treatment of the primary and regional lymphatics. Cancer 34: 156–160

Houghton AL, Robinson MR, Smith PH (1977) Melphalan in advanced prostatic cancer: A pilot study. Cancer Treat Rep 61: 923–924

Housepian JA, Byar DP (1976) VACURG: Carcinoma of the prostate: Correlation between radiologic quantitation of metastases and patient survival. Urology 6: 11–16

Ihde D, Bunn P, Cohen M, et al. (1978) Combination chemotherapy in metastatic carcinoma of the prostate: Method of detecting tumor response and progression. Proc AACR/ASCO 19: 339

Ishihe T, Isui T, Nahira H (1974) Prognosis usefulness of serum acid phosphatase levels in carcinoma of the prostate. J Urol 112: 237–240

Izbecki R, Amer M, Al-Sarraf MA (1978) A prospective study of a combination of adriamycin and cytoxan in the treatment of patients with advanced prostatic cancer. Proc AACR/ASCO 19: 312

Jewett HJ (1975) The present status of radical prostatectomy for stage A and B prostatic cancer. Urol Clin North Am 2: 105–124

Jewett HJ, Eggleston JC, Yawn DH (1972) Radical prostatectomy in the management of carcinoma of the prostate: Probable causes of some therapeutic failures. J Urol 107: 1034–1040

Johnson DE, Scott WW, Gibbons RP, et al. (1976) Clinical significance of serum acid phosphatase levels in advanced prostatic carcinoma. Urology 8: 123–126

Jonsson G, Hogberg B (1971) Treatment of advanced prostatic carcinoma with Estracyt. Scand J Urol Nephrol 5: 103–107

Kadohama N, Kirdani RY, Murphy GP, et al. (1978) Estramustine phosphate: Metabolic aspects related to its action in prostatic cancer. J Urol 119: 235–239

Kane RD, Stocks LH, Paulson DF (1977) Multiple-drug chemotherapy regimen for patients with hormonally unresponsive carcinoma of the prostate: A preliminary report. J Urol 117: 467–471

Kennealey G, March J, Welch D, et al. (1978) Treatment of advanced carcinoma of the prostate with estramustine plus 5-FU. Proc AACR/ASCO 19: 394

Kent JR, Bishoff AJ, Arduino LJ (1973) Estrogen dosage and suppression of testosterone levels in patients with prostatic carcinoma. J Urol 109: 858–860

Klein LA (1979) Medical progress: Prostatic carcinoma. N Eng J Med 300: 824–833

Labess M (1952) Occult carcinoma in clinically benign hypertrophy of the prostate: A pathological and clinical study. J Urol 68: 893–896

Lerner H, Malloy T (1977) Hydroxyurea in stage D carcinoma of prostate. Urol 1: 35–38

Lindberg B (1972) Treatment of rapidly progressing prostatic carcinoma with estracyt. J Urol 108: 303–306

Mackler MA, Liberti JP, Smith MJV, et al. (1972) The effect of orchiectomy and various doses of stilbestrol of plasma testosterone levels in patients with carcinoma of the prostate. Invest Urol 9: 423

McCullough DL, Leadbetter WF (1972) Radical pelvic surgery for locally extensive carcinoma of the prostate. J Urol 108: 939–943

Merrin C (1978a) Preliminary report on combination chemotherapy for advanced prostatic carcinoma. Cancer Treat Rep 61: 313–315

Merrin C (1978b) Treatment of advanced carcinoma of the prostate (stage D) with infusion of cis-diamminedichloroplatinum (II NSC 119875): A pilot study. J Urol 119: 522–524

Merrin C, Beckley S (1979) The treatment of estrogen-resistant stage D carcinoma of the prostate with cis-diamminedichloroplatinum. Urology 13: 256–272

Merrin C, Etra W, Wajsman Z, et al. (1976) Chemotherapy of advanced carcinoma of the prostate with 5-fluorouracil, cyclophosphamide and adriamycin. J Urol 115: 86–88

Mittelman A, Shukla SK, Welvaar TK, et al. (1975) Oral estramustine phosphate in the treatment of advanced stage D carcinoma of the prostate. Cancer Treat Rep 59: 219–223

Mittelman A, Shukla SK, Murphy GP (1976) Extended therapy of stage D carcinoma of the prostate with oral extramustine phosphate. J Urol 115: 409–412

Muntzing J, Shukla SK, Chu TM, et al. (1974) Pharmacoclinical study of oral estramustine phosphate (ESTRACYT) in advanced carcinoma of the prostate. Invest Urol 12: 65–68

Murphy G, Gibbons R, Johnson D, et al. (1977) A comparison of estramustine phosphate and streptozotocin in patients with advanced prostatic carcinoma who have had extensive irradiation. J Urol 118: 288

Nagel R, Kollin CP (1976) Treatment of advanced carcinoma of the prostate with estramustine phosphate. J Urol 115: 406–408

Nagel R, Kollin CP (1977) Treatment of advanced carcinoma of the prostate with estramustine phosphate. Br J Urol 49: 73–79

Nesbit RM, Plumb RT (1946) Prostatic carcinoma: A follow-up on 795 patients treated prior to the endocrine era and a comparison of survival rates between these and patients treated by endocrine therapy. Surgery 20: 263–272

Nilsson T, Jonsson G (1975) Clinical results with estramustine phosphate: A comparison of intravenous and oral preparations. Cancer Chemother Rep 59: 229–232

O'Bryan RM, Baker LH, Gottlieb JE, et al. (1977) Dose response evaluation of adriamycin in human neoplasia. Cancer 39: 1940–1948

Paulson D, Berry W, Walker A, et al. (1978) Multiagent chemotherapy in advanced prostatic cancer — Measurement of response. AACR/ASCO 19: 325

Perloff M, Ohnuma T, Holland JF, et al. (1977) Adriamycin (ADM) and diamminedichloroplatinum (DDP) in advanced prostatic carcinoma (PC). Proc AACR/ASCO C-265: 333

Pontes JE, Choe BK, Rose NR, et al. (1978) Bone marrow acid phosphatase in staging of prostatic cancer: How reliable is it? J Urol 119: 772–776

Ray GR, Cassady JR, Bagshaw MA (1973) Definitive radiation therapy of carcinoma of the prostate. Radiology 106: 407–418

Rubin P (1969) The detection of occult metastatic cancer by radioactive bone scans. JAMA 210: 1079–1080

Schaffer DL, Pendergrass HP (1976) Comparison of enzyme, clinical, radiographic and radionuclide methods of detecting bone metastases from carcinoma of the prostate. Radiology 121: 431–434

Schmidt JD, Johnson DE, Scott WW, et al. (1976) Chemotherapy of advanced prostatic cancer: Evaluation of response parameters. Urology 6: 602–610

Schmidt JD, Scott WW, Gibbons RP, et al. (1979) Comparison of procarbazine, imidazole carboxamide and cyclophosphamide in relapsing patients with advanced carcinoma of the prostate. J Urol 121: 185–189

Schroeder FH, Belt E (1975) Carcinoma of the prostate: A study of 213 patients with stage C tumors treated by total perineal prostatectomy. J Urol 114: 257–260

Scott W, Johnson DE, Schmidt JE, et al. (1967) Chemotherapy of advanced prostatic carcinoma with cyclophosphamide or 5-fluorouracil: Results of First National Randomized Study. J Urol 114: 909–911

Scott WW, Gibbons RP, Johnson DE, et al. (1975) Comparison of 5-fluorouracil (NSC-019893) and cyclophosphamide (NSC-026271) in patients with advanced carcinoma of the prostate. Cancer Chemother Rep 59: 195–201

Scott WW, Gibbons RP, Johnson DE, et al. (1976) The continued evaluation of chemotherapy in patients with advanced carcinoma of the prostate. J Urol 116: 211–213

Shearer RJ, Hendry WF, Sommerville IF, Ferguson JD (1973) Plasma testosterone; an accurate monitor of hormone treatment in prostatic cancer. Br J Urol 45: 668–677

Slavik M, Carter SK (1970) Single agents in prostatic cancer — A quick review. National Cancer Institute Departmental Memorandum

Tejada F, Broder LE, Cohen MJ, et al. (1977a) Treatment of metastatic prostatic cancer with 5-fluorouracil (5-FU) versus 1-(2-chloroethyl)-3-cyclohexyl-1-nitrosourea (CCNU). (Abstract) Proc AACR/ASCO C-10: 269

Tejada F, Eisenberger MA, Broder LA, et al. (1977b) 5-fluorouracil versus CCNU in the treatment of metastatic prostatic cancer. Cancer Treat Rep 61: 1589–1590

Third National Cancer Survey (1974) Advanced three-year report (DHEW National Institutes of Health, Bethesda (DHEW publication no. [NIH] 74-637)

Van Amburg AL, Presant G, Klahr C (1979) Chemotherapy of advanced prostatic cancer with adriamycin (A), BCNU (B) and cyclophosphamide (C). Proc AACR/ASCO 20: 321, C-126

Veterans Administration Cooperative Urological Research Group (1967) Carcinoma of the prostate: Treatment comparisons. J Urol 98: 516–522

VonHoff DD, Rozencweig M, Slavik M, et al. (1977) Estramustine phosphate: A specific chemotherapeutic agent. J Urol 117: 464–466

Whitmore WF Jr (1956) Hormone therapy in prostatic cancer. Am J Med 21: 697–713

Whitmore WF Jr (1963) The rationale and results of ablative surgery for prostatic cancer. Cancer 16: 1119–1132

Whitmore WF Jr, MacKenzie AR (1959) Experience with various operative procedures for the total excision of prostatic cancer. Cancer 12: 396–405

Whitmore WF Jr, Hilaris B, Grabstald H, et al. (1974) Implantation of ^{125}I in prostatic cancer. Surg Clin North Am 54: 887–895

Woodward HQ (1952) Factors leading to elevations in serum acid glycerophosphatase. Cancer 5: 236–241

Yam LT (1974) Clinical significance of the human acid phosphatases: A review. Am J Med 56: 604–616

Chapter 8

Penile Cancer: Natural History and Therapy

R. B. Sklaroff and A. Yagoda

Natural History

Squamous cell carcinoma of the penis although uncommon in the United States and European countries is a significant world health problem. The etiology of penile cancer is unknown, but societies that practice early circumcision and enjoy socio-economic statuses which permit proper hygiene have a distinctly lower incidence (DeKernion and Persky 1978).

Frequently, patients ignore small local lesions on the glans, prepuce, and shaft of the penis and eventually seek physicians' advice when large fungating, infected tumors and inguinal adenopathy are present. However, the presence of enlarged inguinal nodes may not be indicative of tumor dissemination since in half of the cases biopsy of such nodes reveals only reactive lymphadenitis, probably secondary to local infection. Most patients achieve cure by surgery and/or radiation with or without regional therapy since dissemination is relatively late. The primary route of metastasis is via the inguinal lymphatics to the inguinal, iliac and aortic nodes. Hematogenous tumor dissemination occurs to lungs and bone. Death in some advanced cases is the result of hypercalcemia sometimes secondary to production of parathormone-like material. Sudden death may occur from rupture of the femoral artery secondary to local ulceration and necrosis in the groin regions.

Staging

A retrospective review of 135 patients treated at Memorial Sloan-Kettering Cancer Center (MSKCC) from 1969 to 1979 for invasive epidermoid penile carcinoma demonstrated that the great majority of patients presented clinically with local or regional disease for which surgery proved effective. The modified clinical staging system of Hasson (Murrel and Williams 1965) was employed: stage I tumors were localized to the penis without demonstrable lymph node metastases; stage II tumors were localized to the penis with clinically positive operable lymph node metastases;

Supported in part by Public Health Service Grant No. CA-05826 and contract No. 1-CM-57043 (Division of Cancer Treatment) from the National Cancer Institute, National Institutes of Health, Department of Medicine, Education, and Welfare.

stage III tumors were localized to the penis with clinically positive inoperable lymph node metastases; and stage IV tumors indicated metastases beyond the inguinal region to perineum, liver, lung, bone, heart, skin or brain.

The clinical stage of patients at presentation correlated with the incidence of recurrent disease within 2 years of initial therapy and with overall survival (Fig. 8.1). Similar results have been noted by Ichikawa (1977). Clinical and pathologic stage do not always coincide since in 50% of cases, *clinically* palpable inguinal lymph nodes (stage II) have no tumor and patients are thus 'down-staged' pathologically to stage I. It is of note that patients who have lymphadenectomy for stage I penile cancer rarely have a postoperative change in stage.

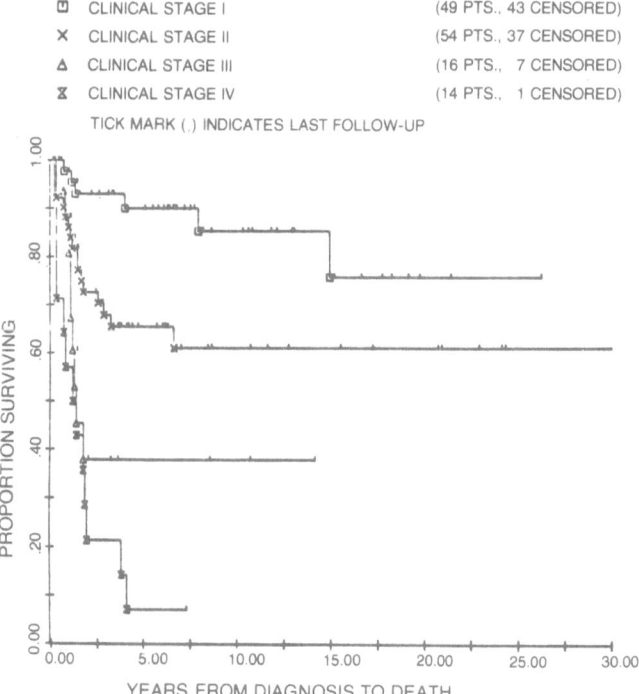

Fig. 8.1. Invasive penile cancer study (MSKCC 1935–1979) — survival by clinical stage.

Investigation

In the initial evaluation all patients should have a screening biochemical profile which includes liver function tests, serum calcium determination and radiographs of the chest and pelvis. In the Memorial series, pulmonary metastases or abnormally elevated serum calcium levels were often detected simultaneously and associated with the presence of inguinal adenopathy (Table 8.1). Chest radiographs were evaluated in 119 patients; seven were abnormal initially and ten subsequently (two of the latter were probably due to a primary lung tumor). Hypercalcemia was noted in 17 of 81 patients tested. In some cases there was no evidence of osseous metastases

Table 8.1.   Correlation of abnormal findings in diagnosis — MSKCC series

	Inguinal adenopathy clinically	Hypercalcemia	Positive chest radiograph	Hepatomegaly clinically	Abnormal liver function tests	Abnormal liver-spleen radionuclide scan
Metastasis on chest X-ray on initial exam	5/7[a]	4/7	–	1/7	2/7	3/5
Metastasis on subsequent exam	8/8	3/7	–	2/8	1/8	0/2
Hypercalcemia on initial exam	10/11	–	4/11	5/11	2/10	2/6
Hypercalcemia on subsequent exam	6/6	–	3/6	1/6	1/6	0/2

[a] Number of patients with positive finding/total number patients tested.

and hypercalcemia was thought to be secondary to a parathormone-like substance (Makoui and Fishbourne 1978).

Diagnostic tests in the Memorial series included radiological skeletal surveys, radionuclide bone scans, intravenous pyelograms, bilateral pedal lymphangiograms and bone marrow aspirations. Of the 29 patients who had a skeletal survey, three who were asymptomatic were found to have erosion of the pubic bone and four cases with known distant metastases elsewhere had osseous lesions. Two of eight patients had an abnormal bone scan. In one case a suspected sacral metastasis and in another a suspected femoral fracture were confirmed. In both cases no other metastases were found. Of 91 patients who had an intravenous urogram, only six were abnormal: three had pelvic disease confirmed terminally and three had non-neoplastic disease. A screening bone marrow aspiration was performed in four patients and none had evidence of tumor. Lymphangiograms were performed in 11 patients and in four, nodal involvement with tumor was confirmed and in only one case was unsuspected pelvic disease discovered. One patient had a negative penile lymphangiogram (Riveros et al. 1965).

Surgery

Partial penectomy is considered the treatment of choice for localized penile lesions. In selected cases a conservative procedure such as circumcision and fulguration has been effective. Carson (1978) used cryosurgery and topical 5FU for verrucous lesions and obtained a complete remission for 3½ years.

In patients with stage I disease only careful observation may be necessary although some investigators have recommended biopsy of the 'sentinel node' in order to determine subsequent therapy (Cabanas 1977). The decision to perform lymphadenectomy should be delayed at least 3 weeks following initial therapy of the primary lesion to allow any inflammation of the inguinal lymph nodes to subside. If the biopsy is positive, a superficial inguinal lymphadenectomy is performed and tumor in the superficial nodes on frozen section necessitates a radical deep inguinal lymph node dissection. Primary lesions which invade the shaft of the penis or the corpora should be managed similarly. However, patients with clinical stage II disease require assessment and treatment of the inguinal nodes. Patients with more advanced disease should be treated with radiation and/or chemotherapy (DeKernion and Persky 1978).

Adjuvant chemotherapy after 'curative' surgery for penile carcinoma has not been adequately studied. Bleomycin was administered with irradiation in one series (Ichikawa 1977) and 8 of 11 patients survived to 5 years. All three deaths occurred within the first year. Four patients given bleomycin and vincristine for stage III and stage IV lesions had sufficient response to permit operation and all but one remained in complete remission for 3+ years (Luciani 1977).

Radiotherapy

Radiation therapy effectively controls the primary lesion in 85% of patients. While the phallus is preserved in most cases, urethral stricture occurs in 31% and eventually penectomy may be required because of radionecrosis (Pointon 1975). Non-randomized trials indicate that the survival of patients treated initially by irradiation is similar to that achieved by surgery (DeKernion and Persky 1978).

Patients with stage II disease who do not respond to radiotherapy may be treated successfully with surgery (Marcial et al. 1962); Orr et al. 1977). There have been no prospective randomized trials comparing the long-term results of surgery alone versus irradiation with subsequent 'salvage' surgery for persistent disease. However, some studies have employed radiation to the inguinal region as an adjuvant to surgery and as a substitute for radical lymphadenectomy for treatment of metastatic disease. In addition, chemotherapy has been combined with radiation therapy. A minor regression for 3+ months was obtained in a patient with metastatic disease after irradiation and 5-fluorouracil (Allaire et al. 1961).

A British group recommends conservative treatment of penile cancer by irradiation, using a plastic mould loaded with iridium[192] (Salaverria et al. 1979). A dose of 6000 rads is delivered to the tumor but only 5000 rads to the urethra. Node dissection was reserved for patients with lymphadenopathy which did not resolve after treatment of the primary tumor. Of 13 patients with stage I or II penile cancer treated with the iridium mould technique, 12 were alive at 5 years, and urethral stricture did not occur. Clearly this technique merits further study.

Chemotherapeutic Agents

Bleomycin

An extensive literature search was carried out to delineate which agents were effective in the treatment of patients with penile cancer. All drug-oriented phase I and II, and all disease-oriented (epidermoid carcinoma) phase II trials were reviewed. The largest series of cases studied was that in Japan (Ichikawa 1976, 1977) with bleomycin, which frequently was used in combination with surgery and radiation as primary therapy for low-stage lesions. Bleomycin was administered in doses of 15–30 units IV or IM, two or three times a week, to a total dose of 300 units. One to three courses were given, at intervals of 2 or more months. However, since the incidence of pulmonary toxicity increased with long-term and high-dose schedules, Ichikawa recommended 'combination treatment of bleomycin with radiotherapy and/or surgery, particularly simultaneous combination treatment of bleomycin with radiotherapy and/or surgery'. Thus, in the largest series of cases only 24 of 188 patients received bleomycin alone and 12 were alive (stage of disease, grade of tumor, and duration of survival were not stated).

Of 13 patients with advanced disease given bleomycin at the Memorial Hospital only one complete and one partial remission were obtained. Responses persisted for only 2 and 4 months, respectively. Bleomycin was given by continuous infusion for 5 consecutive days in a dose of 20 mg/m^2 body surface area. The optimum method for the administration of bleomycin in patients with penile cancer is unknown; patients have responded in all series when it has been given in doses sufficient to produce toxicity (Table 8.2). Data on the use of bleomycin in conjunction with other modalities suggest an enhanced response rate although most patients appear to have had local disease. As a single agent bleomycin may have limited activity against metastatic penile cancer.

Methotrexate

Methotrexate is active against many epidermoid tumors. Sklaroff and Yagoda (1980) reported eight patients with metastatic penile cancer who received methotrexate. One achieved a complete remission following high dose methotrexate (250 mg/m^2 in 4 h) with folinic acid rescue 24 h later. Methotrexate was given for only 4 months and the remission persisted for 11 months. Two other patients achieved a partial remission of 3 months duration with low-dose methotrexate (0.5–1.0–1.5 mg/kg IV weekly). The overall response rate was 38%. Mills (1972) and Conduit et al. (1962) reported responses in patients with penile cancer treated with methotrexate. Although an optimal method for administration (route, dosage, schedule, and associated use of folinic acid rescue) has not yet been defined, methotrexate is effective in the treatment of penile carcinoma.

cis-Platinum

Recent trials with cis-diamminedichlorideplatinumII indicate some activity against penile cancer. Sklaroff and Yagoda (1979) treated nine patients with metastatic penile carcinoma and obtained a complete remission of 7 months duration and two partial responses which persisted for 4 and 2 months, respectively. Merrin (1979) reported partial remission of 2 months duration in two of three patients given cis-platinum. Thus, cis-platinum is active in the treatment of patients with penile carcinoma.

Other Agents

A review of other agents reveals limited trials in patients with penile carcinoma. 5-Fluorouracil produced one minor response in three adequately treated patients

Table 8.2. Results of bleomycin in penile carcinoma

References	Bleomycin Dosage	Route	Schedule	Concomitant treatment	Adequately treated	With metastases	CR	PR	Duration (months)	Bleomycin Total dose
Sklaroff and Yagoda (in press)	10–20 u/m², 10–20 u/m²	IV inf, IV bolus	QD×5d, weekly	–	12	12	1	1	2,4	189, 190 u/m²
Ichikawa (1969, '70, '76, '77)	10–30 u	IM, IV bolus	BIW or TIW	–	59	0	10	29	?	?
Folke (1976	15–30 u	IM	TIW	–	3	1	1	1	48+,5	300, 600 u
Mathe (1970)	10–20 u/m², 20 u/m²	IM, IV, IV	daily, BIW	–	1	0	1	0	–	420 u
Bonadonna (1972)	?	IV	daily or BIW	–	2	?	0	1	–	225–480 u/m²
Ichikawa (1969)	10–30 u	IM, IV	BIW, TIW	S, RT, C	6	1	2	2	–	?
Folke (1970)	15 u	IM	daily	RT	7	0	6	1	6–18	210–300 u
Stephens (1973)	15 u	IM	daily	RT	1	1	0	1	13+	780 u
Abe (1977)	15–30 u	IV	BIW	RT	5	1	5	0	18–82+	150–300 u
Ohnuma (1972)	15 u/m²	IV	BIW	RT	5	1	5	0	–	–
Blum (1973)	15 u	IV	BIW	S, RT	10	0	0	6	–	150 u
Blum (1973)	15 u	IV	BIW	S, RT	6	6	0	4	–	150 u
Luciani (1977)	30 u	IV	daily	S, C	7	4	7	0	36+(×6), <36(×1)	2940 u
Ichikawa (1977)	?	?	?	S, RT	1	0	1	1	6+	310 u

S, surgery; RT, radiation therapy; C, other chemotherapy.

and a minor response in another patient when radiation was administered concomitantly (Brennan et al. 1960; Allaire et al. 1961) Hexamethylmelamine has produced one minor response (Stolinsky et al. 1972). Of two patients with local disease given Coley's toxin, one complete remission occurred which persisted for 5 years (Johnston and Novales 1962; Johnston 1962). There were no responses with hydroxybusulfan, alanine nitrogen mustard and a combination of cyclophosphamide, methotrexate and cytosine arabinoside (Dietrich 1968; Dietrich et al. 1962; Odujinrin et al. 1975).

Primary Melanoma of the Penis

Melanoma accounts for about 1% of malignant tumors of the penile skin (Khezri et al. 1979). In 28 collected cases, the primary site was the glans in 23, prepuce in 4, and the penile shaft in 1. Fourteen patients were treated by partial amputation alone, or in association with block dissection of the inguinal nodes or radiotherapy: no patient survived longer than 2 years. Total amputation, with or without node dissection, was performed in eight patients and four survived 5 years or more. For disseminated disease, chemotherapy is very poor and no agent or regimen can be recommended with confidence for melanoma arising from the penis or any other primary site. The Eastern Cooperative Oncology Group currently is comparing the efficacy of methyl-CCNU with that of methylglyoxalbisguanylhydrazone in an experimental study.

Summary

Surgery and/or radiation therapy remain the primary treatments for penile carcinoma. New techniques which may result in a more accurate evaluation include bipedal and penile lymphography, computerized transaxial tomography of the pelvis, and 'skinny' needle biopsy of abnormal lymph nodes. The initial diagnostic evaluation should always include a serum calcium determination and radiograph of the chest and pelvis. Penile and pedal lymphograms can be used to evaluate the sentinel node and more distant lymphatic drainage. If the sentinel node biopsy contains tumor additional biopsies of deep inguinal and iliac nodes should be performed. If the latter nodes are positive a radical lymph node dissection, sometimes bilaterally, can be curative.

Local lesions can usually be cured by partial penectomy and/or irradiation. All patients who fail irradiation can still achieve cure with partial penectomy. The role of prophylactic radiation therapy is uncertain. In selected cases 'salvage' surgery after radiotherapy has been useful, however, high dose radiation therapy after radical groin dissection generally induces severe incapacitating lymphedema. The role for chemotherapy or limited radiation therapy with or without chemotherapy to enhance operability is questionable.

Bleomycin, methotrexate, and cis-platinum are active single agents against penile carcinoma. Combination regimens still need to be evaluated. In advanced disease methotrexate and cis-platinum can induce partial remissions of limited duration. Phase II trials of other drugs are needed.

The use of chemotherapy prophylactically has not been systematically studied. Bleomycin has been given to 92 patients in conjunction with surgery for penile lesions of unspecified stages; all treatment failures (18) occurred within 2 years postoperatively; and 44 of the remaining 74 patients survived 2–5+ years (Ichikawa 1977). With present data, comparison between patients treated with surgery and adjuvant bleomycin versus surgery alone with respect to disease-free interval or overall survival is impossible. In the absence of controlled trials, adjuvant chemotherapy after 'curative' surgery cannot be recommended.

References

Abe N (1976) Simultaneous combination treatment with bleomycin and radiotherapy for the penile cancer. (Unpublished) Cited in Ichikawa 1976

Allaire FJ, Thieme ET, Corst DR (1961) Cancer chemotherapy with 5-fluorouracil alone and in combination with X-ray therapy. Cancer Chemother Rep 14: 59–75

Blum RH, Carter SK, Agre K (1973) A clinical review of bleomycin — a new antineoplastic agent. Cancer 31: 903–914

Bonadonna G, DeLena M, Monfarini S, Bartoli C, Bajetta E, Beretta G, Fossati-Bellani F (1972) Clinical trials with bleomycin in lymphomas and in solid tumors. Eur J Cancer 8: 205–215

Brennan MJ, Vaitkevicious VK (1960) 5-Fluorouracil in clinical cancer — experience with 155 patients. Cancer Chemother Rep 6: 8–11

Cabanas RM (1977) An approach for the treatment of penile carcinoma. Cancer 39: 456–466

Carson TE (1978) Verrucous carcinoma of the penis: Successful treatment with cryosurgery and topical fluorouracil therapy. Arch Dermatol 114: 1546–1547

Conduit T, Snider I, Owens AH (1962) Studies in the folic acid vitamins: The effects of large doses of amethopterin in patients with cancer. Cancer Res 22: 706–712

DeKernion JB, Persky L (1978) Neoplastic lesions of the penis. In: Skinner D, DeKernion JB (eds) Genitourinary cancer. Saunders, Philadelphia, pp 494–508

Dietrich FS (1968) Clinical trial with dihydroxybusulfan (NSC-390669) Cancer Chemother Rep 52: 603–609

Dietrich FS, Cope C, Rivers S, Krantz S, Baum G, Beck HJ, Rodensky, PL (1962) Clinical trial with alanine mustard. Cancer Chemother Rep 23: 31–38

Folke E (1976) Combined treatment with bleomycin in penile carcinomas. GAN Monogr 19: 231–233

Hofsetter A (1978) Local laser-radiation of a penile carcinoma. Fortschr Med 96: 369–371

Ichikawa T (1976) Studies of bleomycin: Discovery of its clinical effect, combination treatment with bleomycin and radiotherapy, side effects, and long-term survival. GAN Mongr 19: 99–113

Ichikawa T (1977) Chemotherapy of penis carcinoma. In: Grundmann E, Vahlensieck W (eds) Tumors of the male genital system. Springer, Berlin, pp 140–156

Ichikawa T, Nakano I, Hirokawa I (1969) Bleomycin treatment of the tumors of penis and scrotum. J Urol 102: 699–707

Ichikawa T, Nakano I, Hirokawa I (1970) On bleomycin treatment in the urological field. In: Progress in antimicrobial and anti-cancer chemotherapy. Proceedings of the Sixth International Congress of Chemotherapy, vol 2. University Press, Tokyo, pp 304–308

Johnston BJ (1962) Clinical effect of Coley's toxin. 1. A controlled study. Cancer Chemother Rep 21: 19–41

Johnston BJ, Novales ET (1962) Clinical effect of Coley's toxin. II. A seven-year study. Cancer Chemother Rep 21: 43–68

Khezri AA, Dounis A, Roberts JBM (1979) Primary malignant melanoma of the penis. Two cases and a review of the literature. Br J Urol 51: 147–150

Luciani L (1977) Antiblastic chemotherapy and surgical management in the treatment of carcinoma of the penis. Minerva Urol 29: 273–277

Makoui C, Fishburne C (1978) Hypercalcemia in squamous cell carcinoma of the skin. JAMA 239: 1882–1883

Marcial VA, Colon JF, Rojas RAM, Colon JE (1962) Carcinoma of the penis. Radiology 79: 209–220

Mathe G (1970) Study of the clinical efficiency of bleomycin in human cancer. Br Med J ii: 643–645

Merrin CE (1979) Treatment of genitourinary tumors with cis-dichlorodiammine platinum II. Cancer Treat Rep 63: 1579–1584

Mills ED (1972) Intermittent intravenous methotrexate in the treatment of advanced epidermoid carcinoma. S Afr Med J 46: 398–404

Murrel DS, Williams JL (1965) Radiotherapy in the treatment of carcinoma of the penis. Br J Urol 37: 211–218

Odujinrin OO, DeConti RC, Bertino JR (1975) Combination chemotherapy with cyclophosphamide (NSC-26271), cytosine arabinoside (NSC-63878) and methotrexate (NSC-740) in advanced solid tumors. Cancer Chemother Rep 59: 1094–1096

Ohnuma T, Holland JF, Sako K, Shedd DP (1972) Effects of combination therapy with bleomycin (NSC0125066) and dibromodulcitol (NSC-104800) on squamous cell carcinoma in man. Cancer Chemother Rep 56: 652–633

Orr PS, Habeshaw T, Scott R (1977) Carcinoma of the penis: A review of 42 cases. Br J Urol 49: 7333–738

Pointon RCS (1975) External beam therapy. Proc R Soc Med 68: 779

Pow-Sang J (1979) Carcinoma of the penis: Analysis of 192 consecutive cases at the Instituto Nacional de Enfermedades Neoplasicas. Int Adv Surg Oncol 2: 201–221

Riveros M, Garcia R, Cabanas R (1965) Lymphadenography of the dorsal lymphatics of the penis. Cancer 20: 2026–2031

Salaverria JC, Hope-Stone HF, Paris AMI, Molland EA, Blandy JP (1979) Conservative treatment of carcimona of the penis. Br J Urol 51: 32–37

Sklaroff RB, Yagoda A (1979) cis-Diamminedichloride platinum II (DDP) in the treatment of penile carcinoma. Cancer 44: 1563–1565

Sklaroff RB, Yagoda A (1980) Methotrexate in the treatment of penile carcinoma. Cancer 45: 214–216

Sklaroff RB, Yagoda A (to be published) Bleomycin in the treatment of penile carcinoma. Cancer

Stephens FO (1973) Bleomycin — a new approach in cancer chemotherapy. Med J Aust 1: 1277–1283

Stolinsky DC, Bogon DL, Solomon J, Bateman JR (1972) Hexamethylemelamine (NSC-13875) alone and in combination with 5-(3,3-dimethyl-triazeno) imidazole-4-carboxamide (NSC-45388) in the treatment of advanced cancer. Cancer 30: 654–659

The authors wish to acknowledge the secretarial assistance of Mrs. Isa Irvin.

Address for reprints: Alan Yagoda, M.D., 1275 York Ave., New York, N.Y. 10021.

Chapter 9

Primary Carcinomas of the Male and Female Urethra: Other Rare Forms of Urothelial Cancer

B. S. Kasimis

Part A: Primary Carcinoma of the Male Urethra

Introduction

Primary carcinoma of the male urethra is a rare entity comprising less than 1% of all urologic cancers in men (Melicow and Roberts 1978). Thus, no one institution has had the opportunity to collect sufficient data about the natural history, treatment and survival that could be used as general guidelines for the management of patients. Kaplan et al. (1967) collected from the literature a total of 232 cases including 11 patients from their own experience and the Memorial-Sloan Kettering group. Ray et al. (1977) found only 23 cases of primary carcinoma of the male urethra over a period of 30 years extending from 1940 through 1970. Urethral carcinoma is most frequently found in the fifth and sixth decades of life (Kaplan et al. 1967) but in some series where patients with condyloma acuminatum were included, a second peak in the third decade of life was observed (Melicow and Roberts 1978). Generally, it has been noted that urethral carcinoma in contrast to the rest of the urinary tract tumors, appears to favor females more than males (Schellhammer and Grabstald 1978). No racial predisposition has been reported.

Pathology

Like most other neoplasms, the etiology of carcinoma of the male urethra is not known; however, several contributing factors have been suspected. Kaplan et al. (1967) reported that of 232 patients, 37% had a history of venereal disease, 35% had a history of strictures and 7% had a history of trauma. Nonetheless it is unclear that cancer was not present from the beginning in certain case reports of strictures preceding the development of urethral cancer. Mandler and Pool (1966) found no strong association between chronic urethral inflammatory disease and malignancy.

The urethra itself consists only of a mucous membrane supported by a thin submucosal stroma of connective tissue that includes elastic fibers and is enclosed within the corpus spongiosum. Anatomically it is divided into prostatic, membranous, bulbous and penile parts (Fig. 9.A.1). The membranous urethra divides the organ into two segments: the posterior urethra, that includes the prostatic and membranous portions, and the anterior urethra that includes the bulbous and penile areas. The prostatic urethra is lined by transitional epithelium, and the bulbous and penile urethra by stratified columnar epithelium, but the distal penile urethra is lined by stratified squamous epithelium. Hence, different histopathologic varieties of tumors arise, reflecting the histology of the lining epithelium. Cancer of the prostatic urethra comprises 14% of all urethral tumors, and due to its transitional histology, follows the same pattern and shares the same etiologic factors and multifocal nature as tumors of the bladder and ureter. Squamous cell carcinoma commonly occurs in the anterior segment of the urethra. It comprises 77% of all urethral neoplasms and its highest incidence appears to be in the fossa navicularis; adenocarcinoma comprises 7% (Kaplan et al. 1967) and usually occurs in the bulbomembranous urethra arising from the glands of Cowper and Littre, and the lacunae of Morgaagni (Mostofi and Leestman 1971). In order of frequency the bulbomembranous part followed by the penile and prostatic segments are the most commonly involved sections of the male urethra. The majority of the lesions are of low histologic grade. The lymphatic drainage of the urethra shares common channels with the cutaneous, deep penile and prostatic lymphatics. Urethral carcinoma tends to spread mainly by direct extension to adjacent structures.

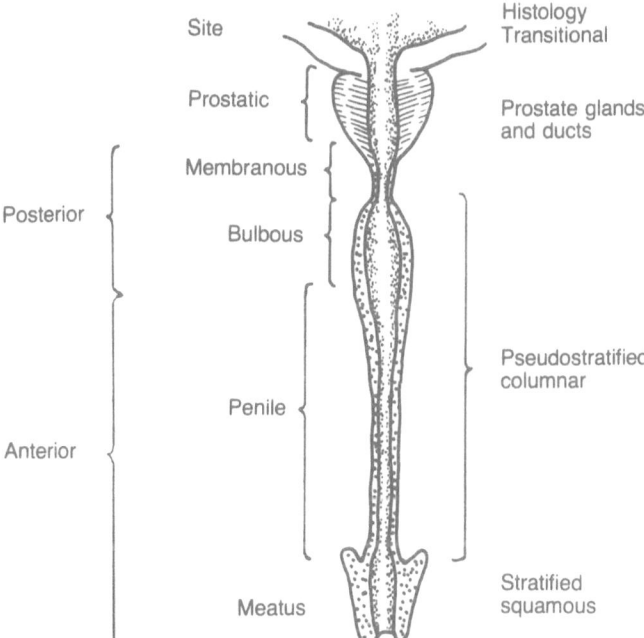

Fig. 9.A.1. Anatomic divisions of the male urethra.

Clinical Presentation and Diagnosis

Commonly, urethral cancer presents as outflow obstruction, palpable mass, peri-urethral abscess, urethral discharge or hematuria, urethral fistula or urinary retention. Uncommon presentations, including palpable inguinal mass, priapism, gangrene and incontinence have been described (Kaplan et al. 1967). Anterior urethral lesions present with a ventral periurethral mass in contrast to posterior urethral lesions which present as perineal masses. Systemic symptoms of malaise, weight loss and fever, usually are associated with advanced disease. Considerable delay in diagnosis, particularly in patients with 'benign' strictures, has been one of the commonest and most frustrating problems that ultimately influences the therapeutic outcome. One should be suspicious in every case where a patient with a chronic urethral stricture suddenly requires more frequent dilatations or develops a urethrocutaneous fistula or abscess. Urethral cancer is easily diagnosed in the majority of cases by a variety of diagnostic tests that include open biopsy, endoscopic evaluation and biopsy, urine cytology, urethral washings for cytology and urethrogram. Lymphography has been moderately successful in delineating pelvic and retroperitoneal nodes. The role of the echogram and CT remains to be determined. Distant metastases at presentation are unusual; thus except where there is definite clinical suspicion, bone and liver scans are of limited value (Schellhammer and Grabstald 1978).

Metastases of urethral carcinoma usually follow the metastatic pattern of the adjoining invaded organs, i.e., prostate, bladder, penis and skin.

Staging

The rarity of urethral carcinoma has been the major factor precluding meaningful statistics. No clinical staging system has met uniform acceptance. However, the following system proposed by Ray et al. (1977) is simple and applicable for the majority of the patients:

O: Confined to mucosa only (in situ)
A: Into but not beyond the lamina propria
B: Into but not beyond substance of corpus spongiosum or into but not beyond the prostate
C: Direct extension into tissues beyond corpus spongiosum (corpora cavernosa, muscle, fat, fascia, skin, direct skeletal involvement) or beyond the prostatic capsule
D_1: Regional metastases including inguinal and/or pelvic lymph nodes (with any primary tumor)
D_2: Distant metastases (with any primary tumor)

The TNM system has also been proposed by certain authors (Schellhammer and Grabstald 1978).

Treatment

Surgical treatment is recommended for the majority of lesions. The treatment plan is usually based upon the anatomic location of the tumor and the existence of metastatic lesions. Life expectancy for the untreated patient is usually less than 1 year. Local tumors of the anterior urethra require partial penectomy whereas radical penile amputation or emasculation have also been proposed. In Kaplan's series there were no local recurrences in patients treated with partial penectomy (Kaplan et al. 1967) and failure to eradicate the disease in rare cases was attributed either to unrecognized lymph node metastases or to the tumors being located more proximally than originally thought. The 5-year survival varies between 50% and 60% (Kaplan et al. 1967; Lower and Hansfeld 1947).

Tumors of the bulbomembranous urethra require total penectomy with en bloc prostatovesiculectomy and cystectomy in an effort to achieve safe surgical margins (Kaplan et al. 1967; Schellhammer and Grabstald 1978). Despite the radical nature of the operation only 13%–27% of the patients survive for 5 years (Kaplan et al. 1967; Ray et al. 1977).

Local lesions of the prostatic urethra have been successfully treated with radical prostatectomy or transurethral resection (Kaplan et al. 1967).

The role of lymph node dissection remains unclear. Most authors agree that inguinal dissection should be contemplated in the presence of palpable inguinal nodes. Pelvic node dissection should follow any radical exenterative procedure for the possibility of removing micrometastatic disease (Ray et al. 1977; Schellhammer and Grabstald 1978). Tumor stage, location and lymph node involvement have a negative correlation with survival (Ray et al. 1977). Radiation therapy either in the form of external beam only, or in combination with radioactive seeds, has generally failed to produce a cure. Rare reports describing long-term control of the disease exist in the literature (Guinn and Ayala 1970; Kaplan et al. 1967). The role of preoperative or postoperative radiation therapy remains uncertain.

Chemotherapy has been practically unexplored in the treatment of urethral carcinoma. Considering the histologic variations of the different urethral segments, agents and combinations known favorably to influence bladder cancer could have the same effect on tumors of the prostatic urethra since they are of transitional cell variety. Agents or combinations active against penile carcinoma could be active against the tumors of squamous histology that arise from the bulbomembranous and penile segments. Local application of triethylene thiphosphoramide (Thiotepa) has been used for superficial or invasive lesions with disappointing results (Cheng and Veenema 1965). However, for patients who refuse surgery, local chemotherapy remains an alternative.

References

Cheng SF, Veenema RJ (1965) Topical application of Thiotepa to penile and urethral tumours. J Urol 94: 259

Guinn GA, Ayala AG (1970) Male urethral cancer: Report of 15 cases including a primary melanoma. J Urol 103: 176

Kaplan GW, Bulkley GJ, Grayhack JT (1967) Carcinoma of the male urethra. J Urol 98: 365–371

Lower WE, Hansfeld KF (1947) Primary carcinoma of the male urethra. Report of ten cases. J Urol 58: 192–206

Mandler JI, Pool TL (1966) Primary carcinoma of the male urethra. J Urol 96: 67

Melicow MM, Roberts TW (1978) Pathology and natural history of urethral tumours in males: Review of 142 cases. Urology 11: 83–89

Mostofi FK, Leestman JE (1971) Lower urinary tract and male genitalia. Urethral malignant tumours. In: Anderson's Pathology, vol 1. Mosby, St Louis, p 856

Ray B, Canto AR, Whitmore WF Jr (1977) Experience with primary carcinoma of the male urethra. J Urol 117: 591–594

Schellhammer PF, Grabstald H (1978) Tumours of the male urethra. In: Cambell's Urology, vol 2. Saunders, Philadelphia London Toronto, pp 1191–1199

Part B: Primary Carcinoma of the Female Urethra

Introduction

Primary carcinoma of the female urethra is relatively rare, but two to three times as common as its male counterpart. McCrea (1952) in an extensive review of the literature found a total of 564 cases and almost 500 additional cases have been reported since. No single institution has had a series large enough to create meaningful statistical data. Although no age group is spared, the peak incidence occurs in the fifth and sixth decades of life. A high frequency among white females has been well documented in several series (Bracken et al. 1976; Grabstald et al. 1966, Roberts and Melicow 1977).

Pathology

Several contributing factors in the pathogenesis of female urethral carcinoma have been suspected. The disease has been described most often in married women, most of whom are parous, while diverticula, leukoplakia, caruncle and chronic urethral inflammatory disease have also been implicated as predisposing factors by several authors.

The female urethra is divided into the anterior segment that occupies the distal third and proximal segment that accounts for the remaining two-thirds of the total urethral length (Fig. 9.B.1). The lining epithelium of both the urethra and the peri-urethral ducts is of the stratified squamous variety, whereas the intrapelvic segment of the proximal urethra is covered by the transitional cell type.

The tumors are classified as 'anterior' in location when they occupy the distal third of the urethra or 'entire' if more than one-third of the organ is involved. The distal third lymphatics drain to the groin nodes but those of the proximal part, to the internal iliac lymph node chain.

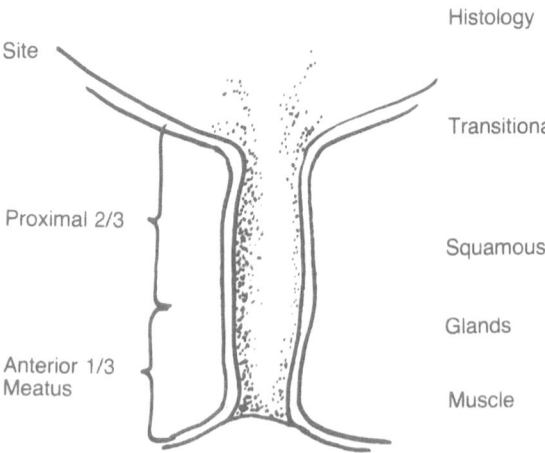

Fig. 9.B.1.   Anatomic divisions of the female urethra.

Epidermoid carcinoma accounts for 75% of urethral tumors; the remainder are adenocarcinomas, transitional cell carcinomas, melanomas, hemangiomas, or sarcomas (Grabstald et al. 1966). The geographic frequency of distribution is debatable. Roberts and Melicow (1977) reported the three predominant histological types to be present in the distal third and proximal urethra, while Grabstald et al. (1966) found no transitional cell tumors arising from any segment.

It is generally accepted that primary adenocarcinomas of the female urethra are neoplasms of the paraurethral glands (Tiltman 1975), while the transitional and epidermoid varieties reflect the pattern of the lining epithelium. Certain tumors arising at the urethrovulvar junction comprise a mixture of urothelial and squamous cells; simultaneous development of squamous cell carcinoma with adenocarcinoma has also been described. As in the case of the male urethra, transitional cell carcinoma is considered to be part of a generalized neoplastic diathesis of the entire urothelium; therefore, the possibility of synchronous or metachronous multiple tumor development requires constant alertness by the physician.

Female urethral tumors tend to invade the adjacent organs and remain localized for long periods before lymph nodes or distant organs are involved.

Clinical Presentation and Diagnosis

Urethral bleeding or spotting is the most common presenting symptom followed by urinary obstructive symptoms, dysuria, urinary frequency, a mass at the introitus, perineal pain, hematuria, urinary incontinence, dyspareunia and urethro-vaginal fistula. Initially the process is well localized. It usually begins as a small papilloma protruding above the surface, or mucosal thickening and induration, or irregular superficially spreading ulceration. In later stages, a fungating mass that bleeds easily is usually present. Adenocarcinomas can present as a polypoid mass protruding from the meatus (Bracken et al. 1976; Grabstald et al. 1966; Fagan and Hertig 1955; Roberts and Melicow 1977).

Palpable inguinal lymph nodes usually are a manifestation of advanced stage disease and have been found in less than 20% of patients at presentation. A detailed physical examination, endoscopic evaluation and biopsy, urine cytology, urethral washings for cytology, excretory urogram and urethrogram are necessary to establish the diagnosis and evaluate the extent of the disease. Although significant controversy surrounds the use of lymphography, it is appropriate to carry out routine pedal lymphograms in all patients as part of the staging procedure (Bracken et al. 1976). The role of the echogram and CT is uncertain. Distant metastases at presentation are rare, and unless there is clinical suspicion, bone and liver scans are of limited value.

Common metastatic sites are the inguinal and pelvic lymph nodes. Distant metastases to parenchymal organs are usually associated with advanced disease stage and occur in less than 20% of the patients.

Staging

Grabstald et al. (1966) described the following staging system, which is applicable to the majority of cases (Bracken et al. 1976).

Stage O — In situ (limited to mucosa)
Stage A — Submucosal (not beyond submucosa)
Stage B — Muscular (infiltrating periurethral muscle)
Stage C — Periurethral
  1. Infiltrating muscular wall of vagina
  2. Infiltrating muscular wall of vagina with invasion of vaginal mucosa
  3. Infiltrating other adjacent structures such as bladder, labia, clitoris
Stage D — Metastasis
  1. Inguinal lymph nodes
  2. Pelvic lymph nodes below aortic bifurcation
  3. Lymph nodes above aortic bifurcation
  4. Distant

Treatment

Although surgery remains the basic treatment, recent advances in planning and equipment have made radiation therapy an attractive alternative for a significant number of patients. However, the rarity of the disease once again has been the major obstacle to studies randomized between the two modalities. Most of the cases in the literature have been treated surgically or by outmoded radiation therapy techniques; therefore, no meaningful comparison of survival data can be made.

Generally, local treatment is advised for stages O, A and B of tumors involving the distal third of the urethra, either in the form of partial urethrectomy or radiation therapy that includes interstitial implants sometimes supplemented by external irradiation. For stages C and D1, more radical surgery in the form of anterior exenteration to include the surrounding involved tissues has been suggested. The role of pre- or postoperative radiation therapy and the indications for pelvic lymphadenectomy remain unknown. Radical surgery should also be performed for local recurrences that develop after partial urethrectomy or interstitial radiation therapy (Grabstald et al. 1966).

In contrast to the anterior urethral tumors, most of the neoplasms that involve the proximal segment of the urethra are of high stage and usually accompanied by lymph node involvement. Although radical surgery has been the traditional approach, uniformly dismal results have led certain authors to recommend adjunctive pre- and/or postoperative radiation therapy (Grabstald et al. 1966). Bracken et al. (1976) reported significant correlation between advanced tumor stage, large size, posterior location and short survival whereas no such relationship could be established for tumor histology or grades of differentiation. In their series of 81 patients, the overall 5- and 10-year survival rate was 32% in a population treated by both modalities in various combinations.

Similar to male urethral tumors, a search of the literature covering the period 1965–October 1979, failed to yield any series where chemotherapy had been used as a therapeutic modality. However, agents and combinations known to produce responses in penile and bladder cancer could be of benefit in cases respectively of squamous and transitional cell urethral tumors.

References

Bracken RB, Johnson DE, Miller LS, Ayalla AG, Gomez JJ, Rutledge F (1976) Primary carcinoma of the female urethra. J Urol 116: 188–192
Grabstald H, Hilaris B, Henshke U, Whitmore WF (1966) Cancer of the female urethra. JAMA 197: 113–120
Fagan GE, Hertig AT (1955) Carcinoma of the female urethra. Review of the literature: report of eight cases. Obst Gynecol 6: 1–11
McCrea LE (1952) Malignancy of the female urethra. Urol Surv 2: 85
Roberts TW, Melicow MM (1977) Pathology and natural history of urethral tumors in females. Review of 65 cases. Urology 10: 583–589
Tiltman AJ (1975) Primary adenocarcinoma of the female urethra. J Pathol 117: 97–99

Part C: Other Rare Forms of Urothelial Cancer

Malignant Tumors of the Seminal Vesicles

Primary carcinoma of the seminal vesicle is extremely rare and the total number of reported cases does not exceed 50. Similar histologic features shared by the prostate gland and seminal vesicles make accurate differentiation between cancers arising from these organs extremely difficult for the experienced pathologist. Lazarus (1946) included 23 cases in his review but being unable to separate tumors of the prostate gland and those arising from the seminal vesicle, accepted only 7 cases as being primary; similar difficulties were also encountered by other authors (Dalgaard and Giertsen 1956).

The age distribution follows the pattern of prostatic carcinoma. The usual criterion for acceptance is that of a papillary or anaplastic adenocarcinoma that involves mainly the seminal vesicles. Frequently the tumors are surrounded by a fibrous capsule and invade the adjacent prostate, bladder or contralateral seminal vesicle. Smith et al. (1967) suggested that displacement of the bladder floor by an extravesical mass, without urethral obstruction, is highly suspicious of seminal vesicle carcinoma.

Hematuria, dysuria, frequency and various degrees of obstructive symptoms with or without perineal or groin pain are the usual clinical manifestations. Commonly the symptoms appear late when adjacent organs have already been invaded. Physical examination usually reveals a small fixed mass arising from the seminal vesicle and expanding into the prostate. Endoscopy, excretory urogram, cystogram, vesiculography and biopsy are necessary for establishing the diagnosis and the extent of the disease.

Surgery is the treatment of choice and usually includes excision of the seminal vesicles, bladder and prostate with supravesical urinary diversion. Some responses to anti-androgen therapy have been reported (Rodriguez Kees 1964). The role of radiation therapy and chemotherapy remains unknown. Although some long-term survivors have been reported (Smith et al. 1967) the rarity of cases precludes meaningful survival data.

Mesonephric Carcinoma of the Female Urethra

Mesonephric tumors usually originate in the remnants of the Wolffian or mesonephric duct. Three cases of mesonephric carcinoma of the female urethra have been reported (Altwein et al. 1975; Murayama et al. 1978). The histologic picture is similar to vaginal and ovarian neoplasms of the same origin. The clinical presentation shares common features with other types of female urethral cancer and surgical treatment with or without radiation therapy should be considered. Local application of triethylene thiophosphoramide (thiotepa) has been used unsuccessfully as a local form of treatment by Altwein et al. (1975).

Other uncommon neoplasms of the urogenital tract including rare forms of sarcomas have been reviewed by Murphy and Gaeta (1978).

References

Altwein JE, Schafer R, Hohenfeller R (1975) Mesonephric carcinoma of the female urethra. Eur Urol 1: 248

Dalgaard JB, Giertsen JC (1956) Primary carcinoma of the seminal vesicle. Acta Pathol Microbiol Scand 39: 255

Lazarus JA (1946) Primary tumours of the retrovesical region with special reference to malignant tumours or the seminal vesicles; Report of a case of retrovesical sarcoma. J Urol 55: 190

Murayama T, Komatsu H, Asano M, Tahara M, Nakamura T (1978) Mesonephric adenocarcinoma of the urethra in a woman: Report of a case. J Urol 120: 500

Murphy GP, Gaeta JF (1978) Tumours of testicular adnexal structures and seminal vesicles. In: Campbell's urology, vol II. Sanders, Philadelphia London Toronto, pp 1206–1210

Rodriguez Kees OS (1964) Clinical improvement following estrogenic therapy in a case of primary adenocarcinoma of the seminal vesicle. J Urol 91: 665

Smith BA, Webb EA, Price WE (1967) Carcinoma of the seminal vesicle. J Urol 97: 743

Chapter 10

Chemotherapy of Testicular Cancer

L. H. Einhorn and S. D. Williams

Incidence

Although testicular cancer accounts for only 1% of all malignant tumors in males, it ranks first in incidence of cancer death in the 25–34 year-old age group (Mackay and Sellers 1966). Thus, cancer of the testis has a significant impact on the social, economic, and emotional status of this young population.

Diagnosis

Testicular cancer usually presents as a scrotal mass first noticed by the patient himself. The healthy appearance of the patient belies the serious nature of the neoplasm. The diagnosis is established by a high inguinal orchiectomy. Scrotal orchiectomies or testicular biopsies are to be condemned as this will contaminate the scrotum and lessen the probability of subsequent surgical cure.

Less commonly, germinal neoplasms may be extragonadal, with presentation in the retroperitoneum or mediastinum with normal testes. The urologist should especially be aware of the clinical situation of a young male presenting with a large retroperitoneal mass and normal testes who is found to have an unresectable cancer at laparotomy which is pathologically read as 'undifferentiated carcinoma'. Because germ cell tumors have a high cure rate with chemotherapy, it would be a major error not to recognize the true nature of this neoplasm, and therefore not to institute appropriate chemotherapy. In any young man who presents with such a clinical picture or with an anterior mediastinal mass in the same situation, it is mandatory to obtain a serum alphafetoprotein and beta subunit of human chorionic gonadotropin. If either of these is significantly elevated, it is reasonable to make a presumptive diagnosis of germinal neoplasm and begin appropriate chemotherapy. Extragonadal germ cell neoplasms frequently are more difficult to manage with chemotherapy because they present with a large bulk of disease compared to patients with a testicular primary who present with or subsequently develop metastatic disease.

Histology and Staging

Histologically, testicular cancer is classified as shown in Table 10.1. Although there are other pathological classifications, including the Collins-Pugh classification that is widely used in Britain, we feel that this is the most clinically applicable classification.

Table 10.1.   Histology

Dixon-Moore	Histology
I	Pure seminoma
II	Embryonal, with or without seminoma
III	Teratoma
IV	Teratocarcinoma with embryonal or choriocarcinoma
V	Choriocarcinoma with embryonal carcinoma

It may well be that the only form of classification necessary is to distinguish a pure seminoma from a non-seminomatous testicular cancer. Radiotherapy is the treatment of choice for pure seminoma as this tumor is exquisitely radiosensitive, there is a 90%–95% cure rate with localized disease, and a retroperitoneal node dissection is rarely indicated (Maier et al. 1968). Although the proper therapy for most seminomas is orchiectomy followed by appropriate radiotherapy, a word of caution should be interjected. Patients who have a 'pure seminoma' diagnosed by orchiectomy but who have an elevated alphafetoprotein (AFP) level, have non-seminomatous elements present elsewhere. These patients should not be irradiated, but should be treated as having non-seminomatous cancer. There is considerably more controversy concerning the management of patients with pure seminoma and normal AFP, but with an elevated beta subunit of human chorionic gonadotropin (HCG). It has been our policy to treat such patients as having non-seminomatous testicular cancer if their HCG level is above 100 mIU/ml, and to use radiotherapy for such patients with clinical stage I or stage II disease only if their HCG levels are below 100. This is a very controversial area, and there are no firm data one way or the other, but regardless of the initial management of the patient with pure seminoma and an elevated HCG level, the clinician needs to be aware that these patients, if treated with radiotherapy, must be followed up at close intervals especially with serial HCG levels.

Testicular cancer is staged according to the extent of involvement (Table 10.2).

Table 10.2.   Stage

I — Limited to testis alone
II — Testis and retroperitoneal nodes
III — Supradiaphragmatic involvement

Surgery and Radiotherapy

In the United States, the standard approach for non-seminomatous testicular cancer that is not stage III is to perform an ipsilateral or bilateral retroperitoneal lymphadenectomy (Donohue 1977). It has been standard practice, especially in certain countries in Europe, to utilize radiotherapy instead of retroperitoneal lymphadenectomy for patients with clinical stage I or stage II disease. There is little question that therapeutic results for clinical stage I or for those patients with clinical stage II who have radiographic evidence of retroperitoneal nodal metastases less than 2 cm in diameter are equally good with radiotherapy compared to surgery, and that radiotherapy will not produce the high incidence of sterility routinely seen when a bilateral retroperitoneal lymphadenectomy is performed. However, the question is not only whether radiotherapy is as good as surgery for primary treatment of testicular cancer, but in this modern era of chemotherapy, we also must ask: 'Is radiotherapy the most appropriate form of treatment for such patients?' As mentioned above, although radiotherapy produces equivalent therapeutic results, there is a major difference in treating a patient with clinical stage I or stage II disease who subsequently relapses with stage III disease and requires chemotherapy if that patient has had radiotherapy. Such patients are extremely difficult to treat: their pelvic radiotherapy hinders subsequent chemotherapy because of severe and prolonged myelosuppression. Also, when drugs such as vinblastine are used in the chemotherapy regimen, injury to the small bowel is considerably more common, and when mediastinal radiation is employed, subsequent bleomycin pneumonitis is likewise more common. These problems are not seen in patients treated with initial retroperitoneal lymphadenectomy. Changes in the philosophy of radiotherapy such that radiation therapy above the diaphragm is not utilized, and that wide pelvic fields are eliminated, would make the above considerations no longer valid. At present, with standard radiotherapy for clinical stage I or stage II, if the patient is not cured with radiotherapy, he is at substantial risk of not being cured with subsequent chemotherapy, whereas patients with clinical stage I or stage II disease who are treated by retroperitoneal lymphadenectomy and who subsequently relapse should have a 95%–100% probability for cure with appropriate chemotherapy.

It is uncertain whether either radiotherapy or lymphadenectomy is needed after orchiectomy in patients with clinical stage I disease (normal HCG, AFP, and normal lymphography and CT of the abdomen, as well as normal chest X-ray and whole-lung tomograms). The only value of radiotherapy or retroperitoneal lymphadenectomy in a patient who has testicular cancer is if there are positive retroperitoneal nodes, as a lymphadenectomy with the removal of 50 or 60 histopathologically uninvolved nodes is of no therapeutic value. Only 15%–20% of patients with clinical stage I disease have positive nodes at laparotomy and retroperitoneal lymphadenectomy. Therefore, in a patient with clinical stage I disease, 80%–85% of the patients will be undergoing inappropriate therapy as orchiectomy alone is all that is necessary.

In the past, even urologists who were aware of these statistics have been legitimately hesitant about not performing retroperitoneal lymphadenectomies, as it was felt that if these patients did harbor microscopically or macroscopically positive retroperitoneal nodes, and if these were not removed, this would seriously reduce the prospects for cure. However, in the modern era of chemotherapy, it is doubtful that this is true, as even if these patients do have involved retroperitoneal nodes, they can be followed closely with a very high likelihood of subsequent cure with chemotherapy or even with retroperitoneal lymphadenectomy. Randomized prospective studies are urgently needed in this area, but patients with clinical stage I non-seminomatous testicular cancer as defined above can legitimately be treated with orchiectomy alone as long as they are followed with physical examination, HCG, alphafetoprotein, and routine chest X-ray once a month for the first year post-orchiectomy and every 2 months for the second year, and then every 3 or 4 months for another 2 years after that. These patients should have abdominal CT scans every 3 months for the first year and every 6 months for the second year. This method of follow-up should guarantee that if the patient was not cured with orchiectomy alone for his clinical stage I disease, metastatic disease should be detected when minimal, a clinical situation which should have close to 100% ultimate salvage rate with appropriate therapy. In clinical trials by the European Organization for the Research and Treatment of Cancer (EORTC), patients with clinical stage I disease are randomized to orchiectomy alone vs. either a lymphadenectomy or radiotherapy, dependent upon which approach is used in the medical center concerned. This is an extremely important study and the results will be very valuable for future recommendations for patients with clinical stage I non-seminomatous testicular cancer.

Chemotherapy

History

Before our present chemotherapy for disseminated testicular cancer is discussed, it is worthwhile reviewing the historical perspectives. In 1960, Li et al. introduced the first major chemotherapy for advanced testicular cancer with a combination of actinomycin-D, chlorambucil, and methotrexate. Subsequent studies confirmed a 50%–70% objective response rate which included 10%–20% complete remissions (MacKenzie 1966). During the past 10 years, several single agents have been shown to possess similar activity, namely vinblastine (Samuels and Howe 1970), mithramycin (Kennedy 1970), and bleomycin (Blum et al. 1973). The major achievement of these earlier studies was not only the demonstration that a complete remission could be obtained in disseminated testicular cancer, but that approximately half of these complete remissions were permanent cures. Furthermore, most patients who relapsed did so within a year of achieving a complete remission with a smaller number of relapses occurring in the second year. Relapses after 2 years of chemotherapy-induced complete remission have been rare. Thus, if a patient with stage III non-seminomatous testicular cancer has been continuously disease-free for 2 years, he is probably cured. Although approximately 50% of these complete remissions were apparent cures, it is expected that modern combination chemotherapy will have a considerably higher cure rate for patients achieving complete remission, because of more effective remission induction therapy with combination chemotherapy which includes cisplatin, and because of increased accuracy in defining complete remission with the availability of radioimmunoassay HCG, AFP, whole-lung tomograms, abdominal CT scan, and abdominal ultrasound.

Of particular interest in these earlier studies was the durability of complete remission induced with mithramycin despite the absence of maintenance therapy (Kennedy 1970). Kennedy utilized mithramycin for 6 months, and then stopped all therapy. It is possible that maintenance therapy is unnecessary in disseminated testicular cancer.

Recent Advances

Combination chemotherapy with vinblastine plus bleomycin was a major improvement (Samuels et al. 1976). Another major advance was the discovery of the activity of cis-diamminedichloroplatinum (cisplatin) in germ cell neoplasms. Cisplatin is one of a group of coordination compounds of platinum that strongly inhibits bacterial replication (Rosenberg et al. 1965). This agent has significant activity in refractory advanced testicular cancer, is the single most active agent in this tumor, and should be part of any combination chemotherapy program for disseminated testicular cancer.

In August 1974, we began a study using cisplatin, vinblastine and bleomycin in disseminated testicular cancer. It was our impression that the best therapeutic results were achieved with vinblastine plus bleomycin and that cisplatin, a highly active and relatively non-myelosuppressive drug, was a logical candidate for addition to that regimen.

Table 10.3. Cisplatin + vinblastine + bleomycin

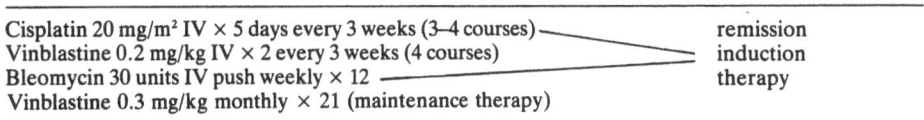

Cisplatin 20 mg/m² IV × 5 days every 3 weeks (3–4 courses)
Vinblastine 0.2 mg/kg IV × 2 every 3 weeks (4 courses)   remission
Bleomycin 30 units IV push weekly × 12   induction
Vinblastine 0.3 mg/kg monthly × 21 (maintenance therapy)   therapy

Fifty patients with germ cell tumors of the testis were entered from August of 1974 through September 1976 (Einhorn and Donohue 1977). Three patients died within 2 weeks of beginning chemotherapy and were considered inevaluable. The therapy regimen is depicted in Table 10.3. Most patients received three courses of cisplatin; however, if a complete remission was not achieved after three courses, a fourth course was given. Vinblastine was initially given 6 h before bleomycin in an attempt to synchronize tumor cells for maximum destruction by bleomycin. However, this kinetic scheduling is no longer felt to be necessary, and we now give vinblastine and bleomycin simultaneously. After completion of the 12 weeks of remission induction, maintenance therapy was given with vinblastine 0.3 mg/kg every 4 weeks for a total of 2 years of chemotherapy. Initially, Bacillus Calmette-Guerin (BCG) immunotherapy was given if complete remission was achieved, in an attempt to augment host cell-mediated immunity and prolong the duration of complete remission. However, the addition of BCG was stopped 3 years ago, and the relapse rate has remained exceedingly low, thus it appears unlikely that BCG contributed any therapeutic advantage.

The primary goal in chemotherapy for testicular cancer is to achieve complete remission and thereby potential cure. Partial remission was not considered a worthwhile goal unless a patient was left with localized disease that could be surgically removed. Of 47 evaluable patients 33 (70%) achieved complete remission (defined as complete disappearance of all clinical, radiographic, and biochemical evidence of disease, including normal whole-lung tomograms, serum HCG and AFP, and normal abdominal CT scans if they were abnormal initially). The remaining 14 patients all achieved a partial remission (greater than 50% decrease of measurable disease). Furthermore, 5 of these 14 patients were rendered disease free following surgical removal of residual localized disease after significant reduction of tumor volume with chemotherapy. The therapeutic results are outlined in Table 10.4. It has been our policy to carry out surgical resection in patients who fail to

Table 10.4.   Results with cisplatin + vinblastine + bleomycin

Evaluable patients	47
Complete remission	33 (70%)
Partial remission	14 (30%)
Disease-free after surgery	5 (11%)
Number alive	31 (66%)
Number continuously NED	26 (55%)
Number presently NED	28 (60%)

NED = no evidence of disease.

achieve a complete remission only if they have residual localized disease. If patients have persistent abdominal *and* pulmonary disease, we have not attempted resection by a thoracoabdominal approach, even though this may be surgically feasible. Also, for patients who present initially with stage III disease, we do not recommend retroperitoneal lymphadenectomy following remission induction chemotherapy unless there is persistent evidence of abdominal disease. In other words, if a patient presents with stage III disease and achieves a chemotherapy-induced complete remission including normalization of abdominal radiographic studies, we do not feel that there is any necessity to perform retroperitoneal lymphadenectomy merely because the patient had no abdominal surgery initially. Instead, we reserve such surgery for patients whose supradiaphragmatic disease is eradicated but who still have radiographic evidence of persistent abdominal disease.

These patients have now been followed up for over 3 years and chemotherapy has been withdrawn in all cases. Four patients died in complete remission in the early part of this study. Two of these deaths were due to Gram-negative sepsis, one from bleomycin-induced pulmonary fibrosis, and one from multiple small bowel fistulae and obstruction secondary to surgery. One of the septic deaths was from *Klebsiella pneumoniae* in a chronic alcoholic who had no evidence of granulocytopenia during this fatal pneumonia. Thus this regimen was directly responsible for two drug-related fatalities.

Only 6 of the 33 patients who attained complete remission have relapsed. Five relapses occurred within 9 months of beginning chemotherapy, and a sixth occurred at 17 months. Furthermore, in all our subsequent experience with chemotherapy of disseminated testicular cancer, relapses after achieving a complete remission always occurred within 1 year of beginning chemotherapy. Thus if a patient with disseminated testicular cancer achieves complete remission and is still in complete remission at the end of 1 year, the probability of cure approaches 100%. Since all of these patients have been followed up for over 3 years, it is highly probable that all are cured, as late relapses were uncommon even with less effective chemotherapy regimens employed in the 1960s.

The relationship of histology to response is shown in Table 10.5. Excellent

Table 10.5.   Histology and response

Histology	No. of pts	% CR
Pure seminoma	4	50
Embryonal (± seminoma)	25	84
Teratoma	2	50
Teratocarcinoma	9	44
Choriocarcinoma	5	60
Yolk sac	2	100

complete remissions were seen in all cell types although there is a suggestion of a higher complete remission rate in embryonal carcinoma. Our subsequent studies have failed to confirm lower complete remission rates in teratocarcinoma, and it is our feeling that all cell types are equally sensitive to this chemotherapeutic regimen.

The most important determinant for achieving complete remission is extent of metastatic disease (Table 10.6). Advanced pulmonary disease was defined as pulmonary metastases greater than 2 cm in dimater and/or more than six pulmonary metastases per lung. Advanced abdominal disease was present if there was a palpable abdominal mass or if hepatic metastases were detected. Nineteen of 22

Table 10.6.   Extent of disease and response

	No. of pts	% CR
A. Minimal pulmonary disease	10	80
B. Advanced pulmonary disease	9	67
C. Minimal abdominal and pulmonary disease	9	88
D. Advanced abdominal disease	16	50
E. Elevated HCG alone	3	100

patients with minimal disease (categories A, C, and E in Table 10.6) achieved complete remission, and one was rendered free of disease after surgical removal of a benign mature teratoma at thoracotomy. The only patients with minimal metastatic disease failing to achieve complete remission all had prior radiotherapy and/or chemotherapy before their initial evaluation at Indiana University.

Radioimmunoassay AFP was elevated in 40% of the patients, and HCG in 75%. Those patients achieving complete remission usually have at least a one log reduction in their marker(s) with each course of cisplatin combination chemotherapy.

The relationship of prior therapy to complete remission is shown in Table 10.7. There was a lower complete remission rate in patients with previous radiotherapy, and as mentioned previously, these patients had considerably more prolonged and severe hematological and gastrointestinal toxicity. We routinely lower the dosage of vinblastine 25% if a patient has had radiotherapy.

Table 10.7.   Prior therapy and response

	No. of pts	% CR
Surgery alone	21	76
Surgery + chemoprophylaxis (actinomycin-D)	9	88
Surgery + chemotherapy (for metastatic disease)	10	70
Surgery + radiotherapy	3	33
Surgery + chemotherapy + radiotherapy	4	25

Toxicity

Although this therapy has produced excellent results, we have been concerned with the toxicity. Cisplatin is potentially nephrotoxic, but this has not been a clinical problem since we routinely employ saline hydration (Einhorn and Donohue 1977). We have not felt a need for mannitol diuresis in any of our patients. Long-term toxicity, especially cisplatin nephrotoxicity, has not been seen and we have not seen any secondary malignancies. Clinically significant bleomycin pulmonary fibrosis also is uncommon. The major serious toxicity has been secondary to high dose (0.4

mg/kg) vinblastine. Myalgias, constipation, and paralytic ileus were all troublesome side effects, but severe granulocytopenia and potential sepsis was the most worrisome toxicity.

Newer Chemotherapy Regimens

In September 1976, we started a randomized prospective trial comparing our standard cisplatin + vinblastine (0.4 mg/kg) + bleomycin (PVB) with the same regimen using a lower dosage (0.3 mg/kg) of vinblastine. Also, because of encouraging results achieved with cisplatin + adriamycin in patients who failed to respond to vinblastine + bleomycin (Einhorn and Williams 1978), a third arm was added to evaluate adriamycin as first-line therapy in combination with cisplatin + vinblastine + bleomycin. The schema for the study is shown in Table 10.8.

Table 10.8. Randomized study of cisplatin + vinblastine + bleomycin (PVB) at two doses of vinblastine and with the addition of adriamycin

R A N D O M I Z E	Cisplatin 20 mg/m^2 × 5 days every 3 weeks (3–4 courses) Bleomycin 30 units IV weekly × 12 Vinblastine 0.4 mg/kg every 3 weeks
	Cisplatin 20 mg/m^2 × 5 days every 3 weeks (3–4 courses) Bleomycin 30 units IV weekly × 12 Vinblastine 0.3 mg/kg every 3 weeks
	Cisplatin 20 mg/m^2 × 5 every 3 weeks (3–4 courses) Bleomycin 30 units IV weekly × 12 Vinblastine 0.2 mg/kg every 3 weeks Adriamycin 50 mg/m^2 every 3 weeks

After completion of 12 weeks of bleomycin, maintenance therapy on all three arms to be vinblastine 0.3 mg/kg monthly for 2 years

Seventy-eight patients entered the study from September 1976 to June 1978, and the minimum follow-up is 18 months. The results are shown in Table 10.9. The complete remission rate (68%) and surgical resection rate for localized residual disease (14%) were remarkably similar to our original cisplatin + vinblastine + bleomycin study. Relapse rate remains low, as only 10 of 64 patients (13%) achieving a disease-free status have relapsed, and again, all relapses occurred within 1 year of beginning chemotherapy. Sixty-five patients (83%) remain alive and 53 (68%) are alive and continuously disease-free.

Table 10.9. PVB ± adriamycin results

	PVB (0.3 mg/kg)	PVB (0.4 mg/kg)	PVB + Adria	Total
No. of patients	27	26	25	78
Complete remission	17 (63%)	18 (69%)	18 (72%)	53 (68%)
NED with surgery	4 (15%)	5 (19%)	2 (8%)	11 (14%)
Partial remissions	6 (22%)	3 (12%)	3 (12%)	12 (15%)
Relapses[a]	2 (10%)	5 (19%)	3 (15%)	10 (13%)
Number alive	22 (81%)	23 (88%)	20 (80%)	65 (83%)
Number continuously NED	18 (67%)	18 (69%)	17 (68%)	53 (68%)

[a] Applies only to those patients in CR or NED with surgery.

Table 10.10. Prior therapy and PVB ± adriamycin

	Numbers	CR	NED + surgery	Presently NED
Surgery alone	52	33 (63%)	9 (17%)	40 (77%)
Prior chemotherapy	17	12 (71%)	1 (6%)	11 (65%)
Prior radiotherapy	15	11 (73%)	1 (7%)	10 (67%)

The effect of previous therapy is shown in Table 10.10. Better results are now achieved in patients with prior radiotherapy. We feel this is because we now proceed with the second and subsequent courses of cisplatin combination chemotherapy *on schedule*, rather than waiting for return of the granulocyte count which otherwise would often delay therapy for several weeks. Thus, the second course of cisplatin + vinblastine + bleomycin is frequently begun when the granulocyte count is less than 1000. Although this greatly increases the possibility of subsequent fever and potential sepsis, we feel this is preferable to delaying therapy and losing the initial therapeutic advantage.

The relationship of histology to response rate is shown in Table 10.11. Although we did not achieve any complete remissions in the six choriocarcinoma patients, three of these patients are disease-free following surgical removal of residual abdominal disease after chemotherapeutic clearing of advanced pulmonary disease.

Once again the most important determinant of complete remission and potential cure is extent of metastatic disease at the time of beginning chemotherapy (Table 10.12). Thirty of 31 patients with minimal metastatic disease (categories A, C, and E) achieved complete remission. This emphasizes the importance of the early detection of metastatic disease, especially in patients who present with stage I or stage II disease and are treated with orchiectomy alone, retroperitoneal lymphadenectomy, or radiotherapy.

The incidence of granulocytopenia with fever requiring hospitalization and the episodes of documented sepsis are shown in Table 10.13.

Table 10.11. PVB ± adriamycin and histology

	Number	CR	NED + surgery	Presently NED
Seminoma	8	6 (75%)	0	6 (75%)
Embryonal	41	31 (76%)	6 (15%)	34 (83%)
Teratocarcinoma	23	16 (70%)	2 (9%)	15 (66%)
Choriocarcinoma	6	0	3 (50%)	3 (50%)

Table 10.12. Extent of disease and PVB ± adriamycin

		Number	CR	NED + surgery	Presently NED
A.	Minimal Pulm	14	13 (93%)	0	11 (79%)
B.	Advanced Pulm	20	10 (50%)	3 (15%)	10 (50%)
C.	Min. Abd. and Pulm	13	13 (100%)	0	11 (85%)
D.	Advanced Abd	23	10 (43%)	8 (35%)	17 (74%)
E.	Elevated Markers only	4	4 (100%)	0	4 (100%)
F.	Miscellaneous[a]	4	3 (75%)	0	3 (75%)

[a] Two patients with cervical nodes only, one with spinal cord compression, and one with bone metastases.

Table 10.13. PVB ± adriamycin and sepsis

	Granulocytopenic fevers	Documented sepsis
PVB (0.3 mg/kg vinblastine)	4 (15%)	0
PVB (0.4 mg/kg vinblastine)	9 (35%)	3 (12%)
PVB + adriamycin	6 (24%)	1 (4%)

Maintenance Chemotherapy

The role of maintenance therapy in disseminated testicular cancer has not been established. In a disease where remission induction therapy is so effective and complete remissions can be defined so accurately, maintenance therapy may be unnecessary. A further aspect of the random prospective study will address this important question as patients achieving complete remission are randomized to receive maintenance vinblastine (0.3 mg/kg once a month for 20 months) or no further therapy after completion of the 12-week remission induction with cisplatin combination chemotherapy.

Summary

One hundred and twenty-five patients with disseminated testicular cancer were treated at Indiana University with cisplatin + vinblastine + bleomycin with a minimum follow-up of 18 months and maximum follow-up of over 5 years. Eighty-six patients (69%) achieved a complete remission, and an additional 16 patients (13%) were rendered disease-free following surgical extirpation of residual localized disease after significant cytoreduction with cisplatin combination chemotherapy. Only 18 of these 102 patients who achieved disease-free status have relapsed; 17 relapses occurred within 1 year of beginning cisplatin combination chemotherapy, and a solitary late relapse at 17 months. Since all patients have been followed up for at least 18 months, we have every reason to believe that we already have the 'final' data on these patients who are free of disease.

A randomized prospective study showed no therapeutic advantage for the higher dose (0.4 mg/kg) vinblastine, and we have therefore dropped this particular arm from our study. We no longer recommend high-dose vinblastine in combination with cisplatin and bleomycin, as we feel that similar results can be achieved with a lower dosage of 0.3 mg/kg of vinblastine in combination with these drugs. The role of adriamycin in first-line therapy is still being investigated.

Historically, our relapse rate has been 18%. In the past 18 months, we have routinely given all patients *four* courses of cisplatin combination chemotherapy rather than our previous policy of giving a fourth course only if there was evidence of residual disease after the first three courses. It is noteworthy that we have had only one relapse of a complete remission patient since we now routinely employ four courses of cisplatin combination chemotherapy. However, the numbers are too small and the follow-up is too brief to be certain that the addition of a fourth course significantly lowers the relapse rate of patients achieving complete remission.

Cisplatin + vinblastine + bleomycin combination chemotherapy consistently produced 70% complete remissions, and a further 10% of patients are rendered disease-free following surgical excision of residual disease. The projected cure rate for patients with disseminated testicular cancer is 70%. Major progress has been made in the past decade as the cure rate for disseminated testicular cancer in the 1960s was less than 10%.

References

Blum RH, Carter S, Agre K (1973) A clinical review of bleomycin — a new antineoplastic agent. Cancer 31: 903–914

Donohue JP (1977) Retroperitoneal lymphadenopathy: The anterior approach including bilateral supra-renal-hilar dissection. Urol Clin N Amer 4: 509–523

Einhorn LH, Donohue JP (1977) cis-Diamminedichloroplatinum, vinblastine, and bleomycin combination chemotherapy in disseminated testicular cancer. Ann Intern Med 87: 293–298

Einhorn LH, Williams SD (1978) Combination chemotherapy with cis-diamminedichloroplatinum and adriamycin in testicular cancer refractory to vinblastine plus bleomycin. Cancer Treat Rep 62: 1351–1353

Kennedy BJ (1970) Mithramycin therapy in advanced testicular neoplasms. Cancer 26: 755–766

Li MC, Whitmore WF, Golby R, Grabstad H (1960) Effects of combined drug therapy on metablastic cancer of the testis. JAMA 174: 145–153

Mackay EN, Sellers AH (1966) A statistical review of malignant testicular tumors based on the experience of the Ontario Cancer Foundation Clinics, 1938–1961. Can Med Assoc J 94: 889–899

Mackenzie AR (1966) Chemotherapy of metastatic testis cancer — results in 154 patients. Cancer 19: 1369–1376

Maier JG, Mittemeyer BT, Sulak (1968) Treatment and prognosis in seminoma of the testis. J Urol 99: 72–78

Rosenberg B, VanCamp L, Krigas T (1965) Inhibition of cell division in E. coli by electrolysis products from a platinum electrode. Nature 205: 678–699

Samuels ML, Howe CD (1970) Vinblastine in the management of testicular cancer. Cancer 25: 1009–1017

Samuels ML, Lanzotti VJ, Holoye PY, Boyle LE, Smith TL, Johnson DE (1976) Combination chemotherapy in germinal cell tumors. Cancer Treat Rev 3: 185–204

Supported in part by PHS Grant MO1 RR00 750-06

Chapter 11

Urological Oncology — A European View

P. H. Smith*

European Organisation for Research on the Treatment of Cancer (EORTC) and its Urological Group

The EORTC was founded in 1962 to stimulate and coordinate research on cancer therapy in Western Europe. Its development has been possible because of continuing financial support from the National Cancer Institute (NCI) in Bethesda. It has also been aided in the last 5 years by private donations collected by the EORTC foundation and, since 1979, has had official support from the European Community.

Its main efforts have been devoted to:

1) screening of potential anticancer agents. This work is complementary to the work in the NCI and almost 4000 new agents are screened annually;

2) the organisation of collaborative research programmes;

3) the initiation of symposia, courses, and publications on the subjects of cancer research and treatment;

4) the development and coordination of cooperative groups to carry out clinical trials aimed at improving the treatment of patients with cancer. Of paramount importance to this role is the activity of the Data Centre.

EORTC Data Centre

The EORTC Data Centre provides statistical advice and monitors the activity of all protocols being undertaken by each of the 15 active cooperative groups. Since its formation in 1974 it has played a key role in the design, implementation and analysis of the studies of the cooperative groups and is regarded by the clinician involved as an invaluable asset. Before any study is undertaken the protocol is designed and developed jointly by the clinicians and the staff of the Data Centre. The final draft is then referred to the Protocol Review Committee, whose membership comes from centres in Europe and the United States. Only after this Committee has approved the concept and design of the study is it accepted for activation by the Data Centre. At

* In collaboration with G. Stoter, R. Sylvester, M. de Pauw and M. Pavone-Macaluso

present 81 protocols are being coordinated (Table 11.1), entry coming from every country in Western Europe.

Table 11.1. Annual rates of entry of patients to EORTC trials (1973–1980)

Year	Institutions	Rand. + registration (patients)	Active protocols
1973	32	332	–
1974	47	496	13
1975	64	733	22
1976	76	1015	31
1977	117	1758	40
1978	158	1779	47
1979	165	2101	63
1980	169	2311	81

EORTC Urological Group

The EORTC Urological Group has existed in its present form since May 1976, when two pre-existing groups, for prostate and bladder, came together. In addition to the Chairman, Secretary and Treasurer, the Group is supported by a National Coordinator in each country, by a Chemotherapy Committee, and by Advisory Panels in Pathology and Radiotherapy. Clinical studies are developed in close cooperation with the Data Centre, the Chemotherapy Committee and the Advisory Panels. The Study Coordinators are selected from those most active in the preparation of the relevant protocols and carry full responsibility for the progress of the trials. In addition to clinical studies the Urological Group has also played a part in sponsoring scientific courses in urological oncology.

In the last 5 years the Group has completed several phase II chemotherapy studies and phase III trials and is currently entering patients in new studies. Each EORTC study has its own code number. The first two digits of each number refer to the cooperative group (EORTC Urological Group = 30) and the second two digits to the year of activation; the last digit gives the number of the protocol in the sequence of those introduced within that year (see Appendix p 149).

Details of the analyses of the completed studies and of the progress in those currently active will be found in sections on the relevant tumours but the general activity of the group can be judged from the fact that members from 12 countries (Table 11.2) have entered almost 1800 patients since 1976 including 344 patients in the 9 months from June 1980 to March 1981.

Table 11.2 List of countries participating in the studies of the EORTC urological group

Austria	Netherlands
Belgium	Norway
Denmark	Spain
Federal Republic of Germany	Switzerland
France	Turkey
Italy	United Kingdom

Cancer of the Bladder

Introduction

Bladder tumours are common throughout Europe but especially so in certain parts of Northern England, where the incidence is up to 24 per 100 000 population per year in men — possibly due to the presence of chemical industries in these areas.

At presentation approximately two-thirds of patients have category T1 lesions, 4–5% category T4 lesions, and the remainder are evenly divided between category T2 and T3, the differentiation between the last two categories being difficult.

In recent years there has been great interest in the development of intravesical and systemic treatments to control or prevent recurrences in patients with category T1 disease, in the evaluation of cytotoxic agents alone and in combination in those with advanced disease in whom primary treatment has failed and who have suitable marker lesions, and in the development of adjuvant therapy for those with category T3 lesions. The EORTC Urological Group has interested itself in each of these categories of clinical research.

Treatment of Recurrent Superficial Tumours

In most areas of the world the treatment of superficial bladder cancer has progressed from open resection and diathermy to TUR or endoscopic fulguration of primary and recurrent tumours. This regimen is satisfactory for the 30% of patients in whom there is no recurrence and for the majority of the 70% who have recurrent tumours. In a few patients, however, recurrences are of such frequency or in such numbers that cystectomy may be felt to be indicated. For these patients at least, it is desirable to develop some alternative treatment. Since tumours arise over many years following hyperplasia, dysplasia and perhaps carcinoma in situ, it is logical to consider local or systemic therapy additional to TUR.

Over the years chemical agents including podophyllin, silver nitrate, radioactive isotopes and many cytotoxic agents have been tried, without conspicuous success (Abbassian and Wallace 1966; Jacobi et al. 1979; Pavone-Macaluso 1979). The use of iridium-192 wiring and of interstitial radium implants has been recommended by Auvert and Botto (1980) and Werf-Messing (1980). In addition bladder distension therapy (Helmstein 1972), mucosal denudation (Lund 1969), treatment with Vitamins A, B_6, and C (Bishop 1980; Byar et al. 1977; Schlegel et al. 1970) and the use of BCG intravesically and by scarification have also found favour (Morales et al. 1976; Douville et al. 1978; Lamm et al. 1980; Martinez-Piñeiro 1980) whilst oral cyclophosphamide and oral methotrexate are also being used in an attempt to control carcinoma in situ and recurrent category T1 lesions (England et al. 1980a; Hall 1980).

The aim of such therapy may be to treat existing tumours, to prevent their recurrence following TUR, or to prevent that progression of stage or grade which occurs in 10–44% of category T1 lesions (England et al. 1980b; Prout 1981).

The EORTC Urological Group has completed one phase III trial of intravesical cytotoxic therapy and is now recruiting to three further studies, two of intravesical chemotherapy and one to evaluate the role of oral pyridoxine. The details of these studies are given in Table 11.3.

In the interim analysis of the first study (Schulman and EORTC Group 1980) intravesical thiotepa has been shown to be superior to VM26 and to no additional treatment following TUR in reducing the incidence of recurrent lesions (Table 11.4)

Table 11.3. EORTC urological group protocols for the treatment of category T1 bladder cancer

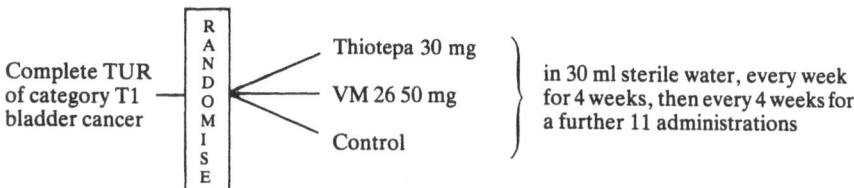

Protocol 30751. A comparison of intravesical thiotepa, VM26 and control. Study Coordinator Dr C.C. Schulman, Brussels, Belgium. Activated November 1975. Closed October 1978 with 294 evaluable patients.

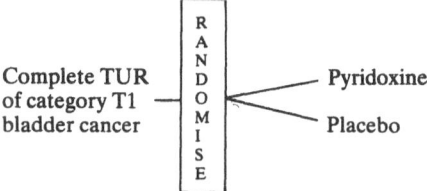

Protocol 30781. A comparison of oral pyridoxine (20 mg/day) and placebo. Study coordinator Mr M.R.G. Robinson, Pontefract, England. 253 patients entered since January 1979. A double blind study with tryptophan load tests before and after 6 months of treatment.

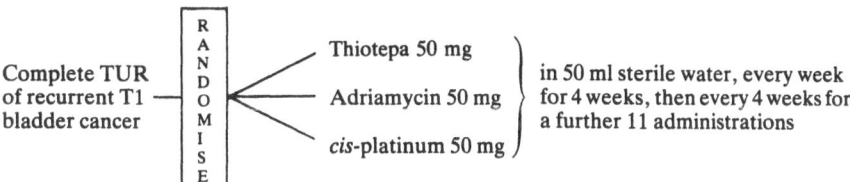

Protocol 30782. A comparison of intravesical thiotepa, adriamycin, and *cis*-platinum. Study Co-ordinators Dr C.C. Schulman, Brussels, Belgium, and Prof. M. Pavone-Macaluso, Palermo, Sicily. 207 patients entered since March 1979.

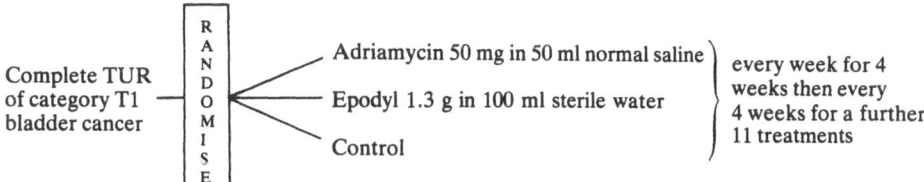

Protocol 30790. A comparison of intravesical adriamycin, epodyl and control. Study Coordinator Dr K. Kurth, Rotterdam, Holland. 141 patients entered since December 1979.

and toxicity has been minimal (Table 11.5). The final analysis of this study is now in preparation.

The EORTC studies in which patients with both primary and recurrent lesions were given chemo-prophylaxis following TUR have made clear that this approach is (1) inconvenient for the patient unless instillation is restricted to the times of check cytoscopy; (2) expensive in terms of drugs (Table 11.6), nursing and medical time;

Table 11.4. EORTC Protocol 30751. Recurrences by treatment (all patients)

	Thiotepa[a]	VM26	No treatment	Total
No. of patients randomised	115	116	109	340
No. of patients with follow-up	75	71	69	215
No. of patients with recurrences	37	44	36	117
Percent with recurrences	49.3	62.0	52.2	54.4
Total no. of recurrences	58	69	68	195
Total months of follow-up	837	682	682	2201
Recurrence rate/100 patient months	6.93	10.12	9.97	8.86

[a] Triethylene thiophosphoramide.

Table 11.5. Toxicity of intravesical thiotepa 30 mg and control in EORTC Protocol 30751

	Thiotepa (89 pts)	Control (82 pts)
WBC < 4500	2	2
Platelets < 150 000	14	10
Hb < 11G	1	2
WBC < 4500 and platelets < 150 000	4	–
Hb < 11 g/litre and WBC < 4500	1	–
Hb < 11 g/litre and platelets < 150 000	–	2
Treatment stopped because of toxicity	3	–

Table 11.6. Cost of some agents used in intravesical therapy

Agent	Sterling	Dollars
Thiotepa 30 mg (15 mg vials)	8.80	17
Epodyl 1.3 gm (1 amp)	2.54	4.90
Adriamycin 50 mg	47.95	93
Mitomycin C 30 mg (2 mg vials)	59.50	115.40

and (3) not necessary unless the patient has recurrent lesions and is clearly indicated only for those with frequent recurrences, which are difficult to control and perhaps for those with carcinoma in situ demonstrated at random biopsy.

Intravesical therapy is usually given weekly or monthly, but Burnand et al. (1976) suggested that instillation only at check cystoscopy was also effective in reducing the incidence of recurrent lesions. This thesis is attractive and is to be studied in a trial developed by the Medical Research Council (MRC) in the United Kingdom in which patients, following complete resection of newly diagnosed Ta/T1 transitional cell bladder cancer, will be randomly allocated to receive:

Thiotepa 30 mg (as soon as possible after TUR)	vs	Thiotepa 30 mg (after TUR and on four subsequent check cystoscopies at 3-monthly intervals)	vs	No additional treatment after TUR

Instillation will be for a period of 1 h after which the drug will be drained from the bladder. The end-point will be the first recurrence after 1 year. If this trial proves that intravesical chemotherapy is effective when given in this way, it will make the whole concept of such treatment much more attractive.

Phase II Studies

Since the original paper of Carter and Wasserman (1975) a great deal of information on the effect of different cytotoxic agents has been obtained from phase II studies in patients with advanced disease who have failed primary treatment. The increasing emphasis on the importance of measurable metastases in such studies has improved the quality of the data but as yet the incidence of remission is rarely in excess of 40% and combination therapy has not been demonstrated to be superior to single agent treatment. Adriamycin (ADM), cisplatin (DDP), cyclophosphamide (CTX), 5-fluorouracil (5-FU), methotrexate (MTX), and mitomycin C have all been shown to be active (Smith 1981a).

Phase II studies are an integral part of the preliminary work which must be undertaken before drugs can be used in the adjuvant situation. The EORTC group has now completed two studies and is recruiting to two more.

In the initial EORTC study of ADM 50 mg/m^2 + 5-FU 500 mg/m^2 3-weekly for at least four cycles, there was a 40% objective response rate with relief of bone pain and haematuria in approximately 50% of patients. The second study, restricted to patients with measurable metastatic lesions and using the combination of CTX, ADM, and DDP, has now been closed to recruitment with 42 evaluable patients. The full analysis of this study is awaiting publication and shows 4 complete and 12 partial remissions, a response rate of 38%, lower than in the initial report by Sternberg et al. (1977). Studies with vincristine and with DDP plus VM26 are in progress.

Adjuvant Chemotherapy in Bladder Cancer

The search for effective chemotherapeutic agents is only necessary because of the unsatisfactory results obtained from conventional primary treatment, whether by cystectomy, radiotherapy or the combination of these modalities in category T3 bladder cancer.

The defects of conventional therapy are well illustrated by the results of the collaborative trial of radical radiotherapy versus preoperative radiotherapy and radical cystectomy (Wallace and Bloom 1976). Despite the fact that patients had to be fit enough to be suitable for cystectomy at the time of randomisation, the subsequent progress in both groups was depressingly unsatisfactory since 40% of patients on both arms of the study were dead within 1 year.

This high early mortality is a feature of category T3 bladder cancer and has led some people to avoid cystectomy as primary treatment (Blandy et al. 1980; Weaver et al. 1979), reserving it for those patients whose tumour persists or recurs after radical radiotherapy. The overall 5-year survival of 38% obtained by Blandy et al. (1980) with this approach is not inferior to that of preoperative radiation followed by cystectomy and also highlights the great difference in survival between those whose tumours are radiosensitive and those in whom no response is seen after radiotherapy (56% vs. 17% crude 5-year survival).

The early mortality, largely due to the patients with radioresistant tumours, is however still high and if this could be controlled by effective adjuvant cytotoxic therapy the outlook for the patient with invasive bladder cancer would be greatly improved.

At least three trials of adjuvant chemotherapy have been activated in different European centres. Of these:

1) The EORTC study (Protocol 30784) was designed to compare the value of adriamycin and 5-fluorouracil against no additional treatment following radical cystectomy with or without preoperative flash radiotherapy (1500 rads in 2 days) for P3 NO-2 MO bladder cancer. Despite initial enthusiasm in many continental centres, recruitment was unsatisfactory and the trial was closed in March 1981.

2) In a study in London and Oxford, patients with T3 NX MO bladder cancer are randomised to receive methotrexate or no additional treatment in addition to their primary therapy. The primary therapy is 4000 rads followed by radical cystectomy for those under 65 years of age, and radical radiotherapy for those over 65, unless it is the policy of the hospital concerned to treat all patients primarily by radiotherapy. Those patients randomised to the chemotherapeutic arm receive three doses of methotrexate at 3-weekly intervals before radiotherapy and the same treatment following completion of their primary treatment, every 2 weeks for 6 months.

3) In the Yorkshire Urological Co-operative Research Group a trial of adriamycin 50 mg/m^2 and 5-fluorouracil 500 mg/m^2 3-weekly versus no additional treatment following radical radiotherapy has been completed. In the 101 evaluable patients the 1-year survival figures are very similar in each arm and statistical evaluation shows that there is a less than 5% chance that there is a 20% difference in survival (Smith 1981a).

Clearly, some time will elapse before adjuvant chemotherapy can be fully assessed. However, several drugs show activity in phase II studies and it should be possible to integrate cytotoxic chemotherapy, radiotherapy and surgery in such a way that survival is improved. From his training the surgeon is always anxious to remove the primary lesion and the radiotherapist to 'sterilise' the area in which the tumour lies. Given the high early death rate and the fact that 35% of patients die with distant metastases (Prout 1977) it may prove necessary to ask surgeons and radiotherapists to adjust their attitudes and to allow the medical oncologist to administer chemotherapy before conventional primary treatment is given. This approach is already being carried out in the London and Oxford study and the early results of this study will therefore be awaited with special interest.

Cancer of the Prostate

Introduction

The challenge presented by cancer of the prostate is still unresolved. Although clinical and histological diagnosis is not difficult, the significance of such a diagnosis, especially in the categories T0–T2, and in all categories in patients over 75 years of age, remains the subject of debate.

The increase in incidence of early diagnosis, as shown by the increase in patients with stage A and B (category T0–T2) disease when routine rectal examinations are carried out (McMillen and Wettlaufer 1976), presents the clinician with a difficult problem since there is no clear evidence that, for such patients, one treatment is superior to another or even to deferred treatment. The 5-year survival following varying therapies in the different stages of this disease is shown in Table 11.7.

The overall survival following such different treatment regimens is so similar and survival between different G (grade) categories so diverse (Heaney et al. 1977; Bagshaw 1982a) that the treatment of choice is not clear and variations in survival in any study which is not randomised and stratified for G category are likely to be due to factors other than the therapy.

Table 11.7. Five-year survival rate by stage after placebo, hormones[a], radiotherapy[b], and radical prostatectomy[c]

Treatment	Veterans stage and percentage 5-year survival			
	A	B	C	D
Placebo	70	70	50	25
Hormones	70	70	50	25
Radiotherapy	80	75	60	–
Radical prostatectomy	80	75	65	–

[a] VACURG 1967.
[b] Bagshaw, to be published.
[c] Boxer et al. 1977; Schroeder and Belt 1975.

Clinical Trials in Europe

Urological surgeons in Europe have become concerned by these unsolved problems. In the United Kingdom the MRC has now implemented two trials designed to obtain further information on the results of treatment in patients with category MO disease, i.e., carcinoma localised to the prostate:

1) In the first trial patients with early cancer of the prostate (category T0–T1 NX MO) are randomised to receive either radiotherapy — 5000 rads in 20 fractions over 4 weeks with a field size not greater than $10 \, cm^3$ — or deferred treatment.

2) In the second trial, patients with category T2–T4 NX MO lesions are randomised between orchiectomy, radiotherapy, and radiotherapy plus orchiectomy. This study is designed to determine whether orchiectomy, radiotherapy, or the combination of these therapies will delay the appearance of metastases and prolong survival.

These studies, begun in 1979 and 1980, respectively, are unlikely to yield any results for at least 4–5 years.

For patients with metastatic disease, the clinical problem is to relieve symptoms, to prevent progression of the disease and if possible to induce objective remission. This problem is unsolved. It is now accepted that oestrogens, orchiectomy and deferred treatment carry their own benefits and hazards but that overall survival is similar (VACURG 1967). The search for alternative hormonal agents and the investigation of combinations of hormonal agents with chemotherapy continues (Beckley et al. 1980; Smith 1980). As yet no form of hormone therapy has been demonstrated to be superior to conventional oestrogen treatment.

In Europe, the EORTC Urological Group has completed two studies to compare stilboestrol (DES) versus estramustine in one study and DES versus cyproterone acetate (CPA) versus medroxyprogesterone acetate (MPA) in the other. The details are shown in Table 11.8.

Although it will be another 3 years at least before these protocols undergo final

Table 11.8.   EORTC Urological Group protocols for the treatment of advanced prostatic cancer

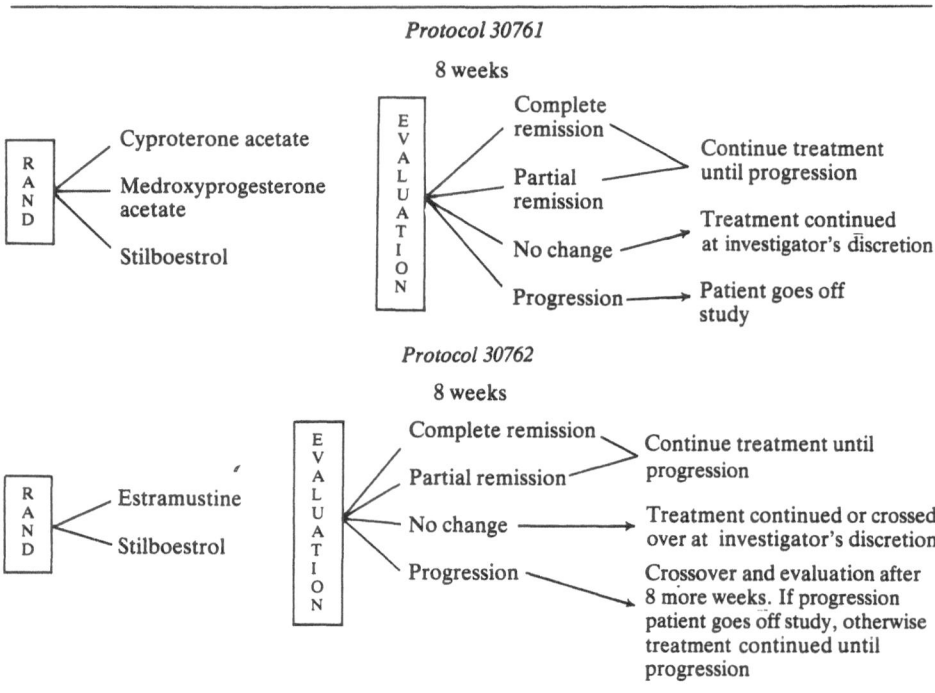

analysis, certain preliminary observations can be made (de Pauw et al. 1982). It appears that:

1) DES 1 mg t.d.s. carries a cardiovascular hazard,

2) MPA at the dose used is inferior to DES and CPA in preventing progression of the disease, and

3) DES and estramustine both produce objective remission of bony metastases, partial or complete, in approximately one third of patients.

The incidence of objective remission is similar to that reported by Beckley et al. (1980) and establishes a reference point against which the combination of hormones and chemotherapy must be judged.

The Group has replaced these studies with a new trial (Protocol 30805) to compare:

DES   vs. Orchiectomy vs. Orchiectomy + CPA
1 mg daily   (50 mg t.d.s.)

for patients with category M1 disease. The orchiectomy may be either total or subcapsular. For patients who refuse orchiectomy and for centres which prefer to avoid it a further study is in preparation. In this alternative protocol it is proposed to compare:

CPA   vs. CPA   + Lisuride
(50 mg t.d.s.)   (50 mg t.d.s.)   (An antiprolactin agent)

Entry will again be restricted to patients with category M1 disease. As a consequence, urologists in the United Kingdom will now have the opportunity to enter all patients with newly diagnosed prostatic cancer into prospectively randomised studies — two being organised by the MRC for patients with disease localised to the prostate and two by the EORTC for patients with metastatic disease.

Cytotoxic Therapy

The place of cytotoxic chemotherapy in cancer of the prostate has yet to be established. The majority of the work on the use of cytotoxic agents in the last few years has come from the National Prostatic Cancer Project (NPCP). In these studies (Beckley et al. 1980), patients who do not show progression and those who have stable disease are grouped with those showing complete or partial remission to form a category of 'objective response'. Unfortunately the high rates of 'objective response' reported in the NPCP studies are largely dependent upon the patients with stable disease. The numbers of partial and complete objective remissions are very few (Smith 1981b) and it seems that the majority of agents so far investigated are relatively inactive, at least in phase II studies in patients with advanced prostatic cancer (Smith 1980).

There is some evidence (Kliman et al. 1978) that 'hormonal escape' in prostatic cancer may be due to the continuing growth of a proportion of cells which have never been hormone-sensitive. If this hypothesis proves to be valid there will be obvious justification for the use of systemic non-hormonal therapy at the time of diagnosis once effective agents become available, of which there is yet little evidence (Smith 1981b).

The association of hormonal and cytotoxic therapy has already been used in NPCP study 500, in which standard therapy is compared to DES plus CTX in one arm and DES plus estramustine in another. The early results of Protocol 500 have recently been reported by Schmidt (1982). Unfortunately there is no evidence of superiority of the arms containing chemotherapy.

Further work is urgently required to identify drugs which are capable of inducing a substantial proportion of partial and complete objective remissions so that other trials of adjuvant chemotherapy may be initiated. As yet the EORTC Urological Group has had little success. Houghton et al. (1977) reported no response in 15 patients treated with melphalan and in EORTC Protocol 30763 in which adriamycin (ADM) or procarbazine (PCB) was given, treatment with PCB had to be stopped because of gastrointestinal intolerance and a high incidence of early death. Only one partial response was seen in 14 patients treated with PCB. The current study (Protocol 30799) is to evaluate vindesine in patients with advanced disease with marker lesions.

Conclusions

Little progress has been made since the first VACURG study was reported in 1967. Oestrogen therapy and orchiectomy remain the mainstays of treatment for the patient with disseminated disease. For the patient with local disease the timing and the choice of therapy are both open questions and are being investigated in the MRC trials, whilst alternatives to oestrogens and orchiectomy are being investigated in the EORTC studies in patients with metastatic disease. Although effective cytotoxic therapy is required, the agents so far tested produce few objective remissions.

Cancer of the Kidney

Introduction

Carcinoma of the kidney is uncommon, forming only 1%–2% of all tumours. As a result the individual urologist sees relatively few cases, perhaps five to ten per year for the majority of those in Europe, with the exception of certain specialised centres.

The kidney is a relatively inaccessible organ and diagnosis of lesions at an early stage is often difficult. Some tumours grow relatively quickly (Fig. 11.1), whilst others change little over a period of years (Fig. 11.2). Even when the patient is seen

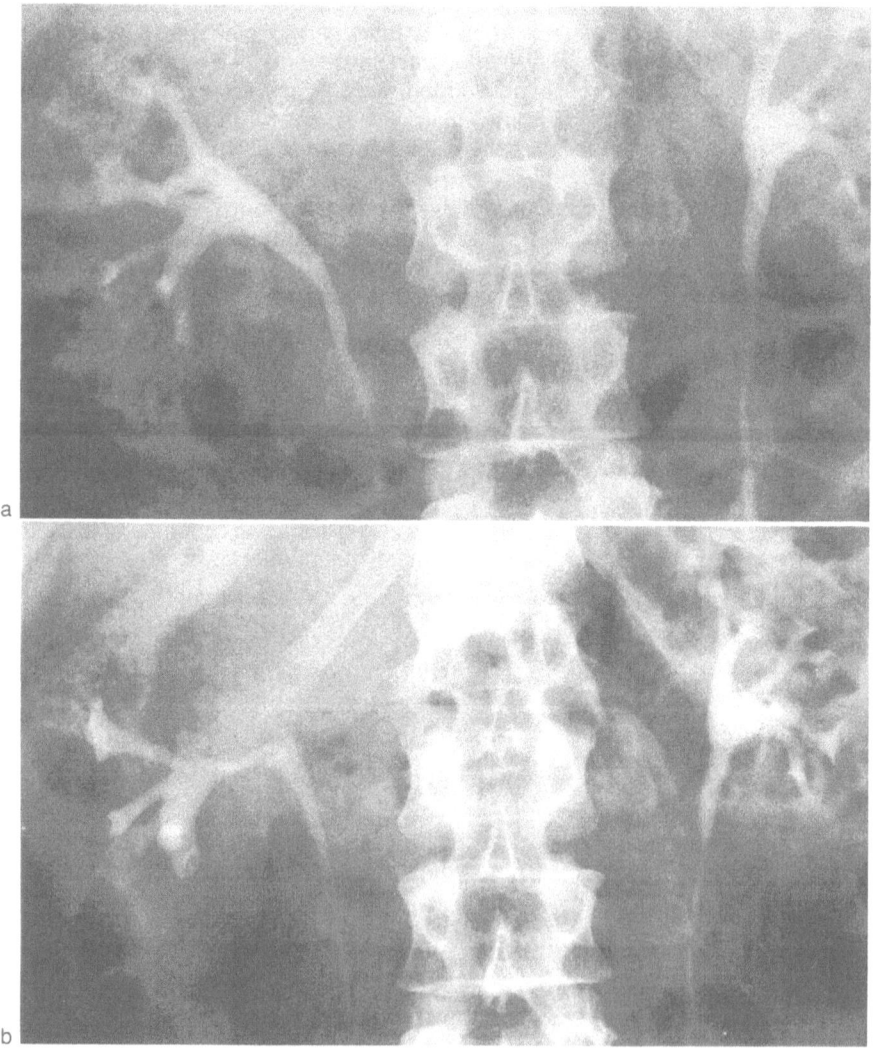

Fig. 11.1. a Intravenous pyelogram of a patient following one episode of haematuria. **b** Repeat pyelogram 5 months later.

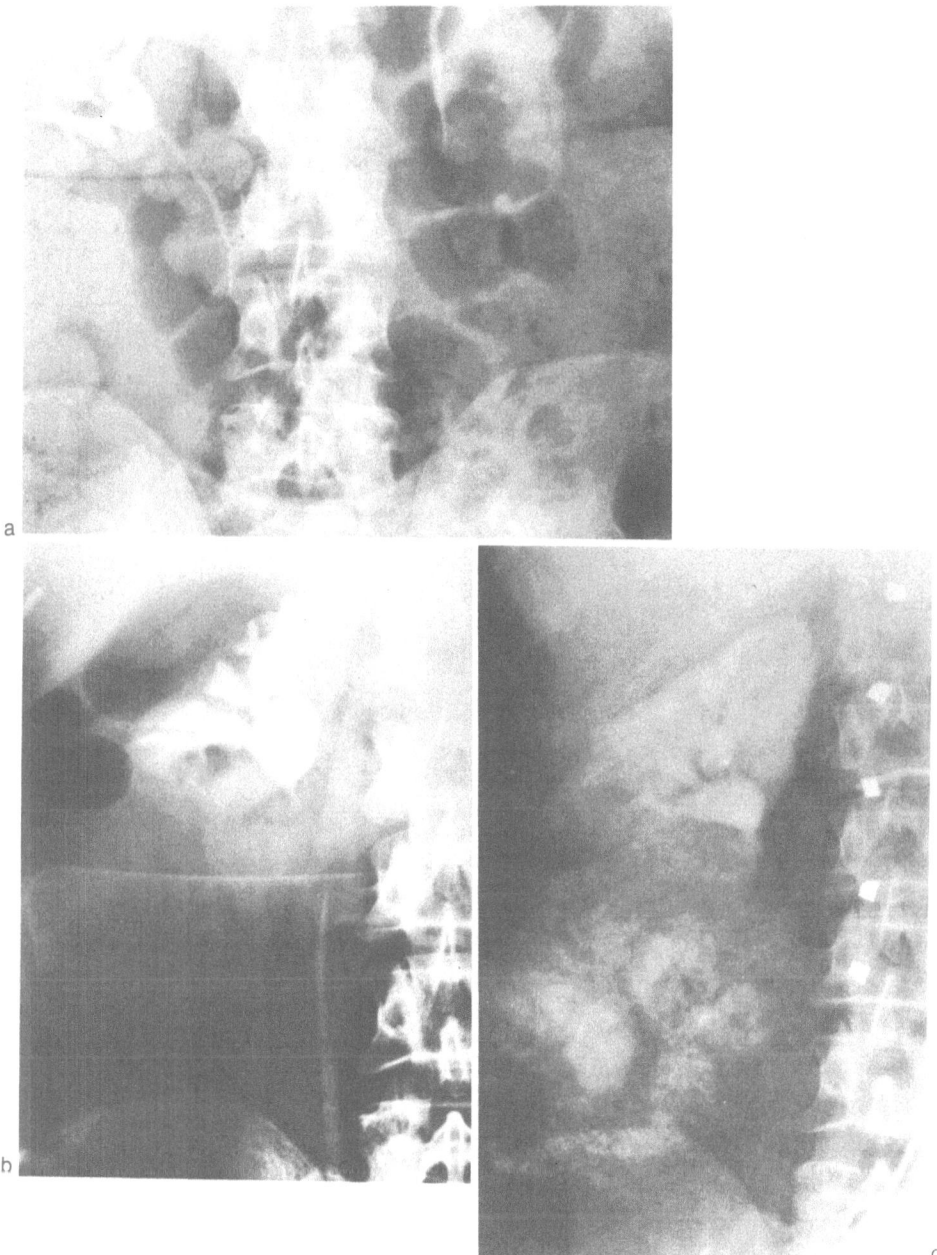

Fig. 11.2. **a** Intravenous pyelogram in hypertensive patient in 1969. **b** Repeat pyelogram in 1971. **c** Angiogram in 1971. The patient had no symptoms referable to the primary tumour.

within 12 h of his first symptom (Fig. 11.3) the lesion may be extensive. Survival is related to both grade and stage and whilst the surgeon cannot influence the grade of a lesion he could offer the patient a better prognosis if the diagnosis could be made at an earlier stage. Unfortunately many patients present only with metastases (Fig. 11.4), having had no symptoms from the primary tumour, whilst in others it is

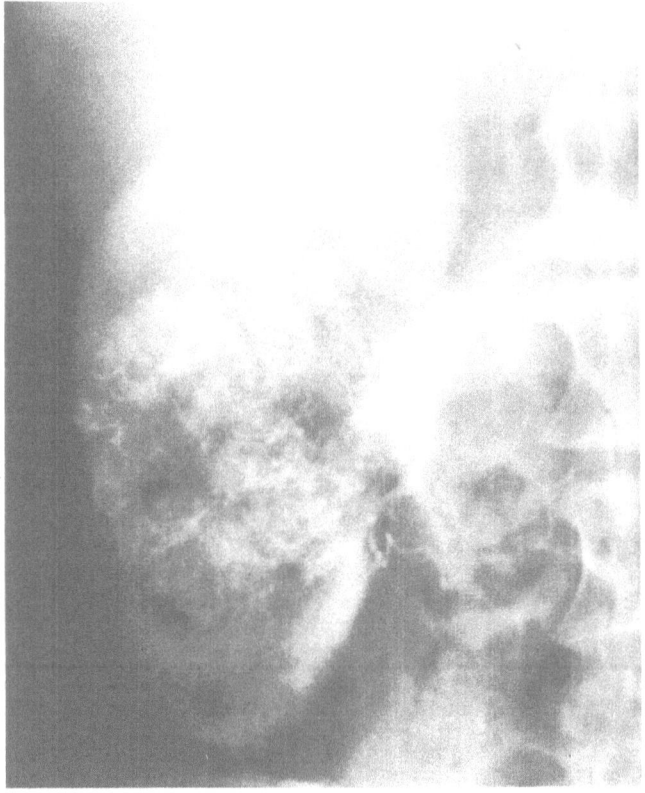

Fig. 11.3. Angiogram of patient 5 days after first episode of haematuria.

symptoms of a general and non-specific nature that make them seek medical advice. A wider understanding in general medical circles of the potential urological importance of a pyrexia of unknown origin, a raised ESR, a raised α-2 globulin and of the paraneoplastic syndromes so well described by Chisholm and Roy (1971) and Altaffer and Chenault (1979) might improve the cure rate and survival time.

Once suspected, the diagnosis is easy to make by intravenous urography with nephrotomography, ultrasound, CT scan and, if necessary, angiography, at which time embolisation may be performed by one of the several techniques available.

The traditional treatment by radical nephrectomy is satisfying to the surgeon but has yet to be proved superior to simple nephrectomy. At a recent NATO Advanced Study Institute meeting the question of lymphadenectomy was reviewed (Carmignani 1982), the emphasis during discussion being that excision of lymph nodes was more a guide to prognosis than an aid to survival, since it was exceedingly unlikely that in patients with involved nodes, other foci of neoplasm would not be present. The results of the Rotterdam renal carcinoma trial are of interest in this regard, since they show high survival rates for simple nephrectomy in category P1 + P2 lesions (60% at 5 years) and a clear relationship between ESR and prognosis (Werf-Messing et al. 1978), suggesting that factors other than extent of surgical excision are of great prognostic importance. In this study half the patients were randomised to receive pre-operative radiotherapy which did not influence the outcome.

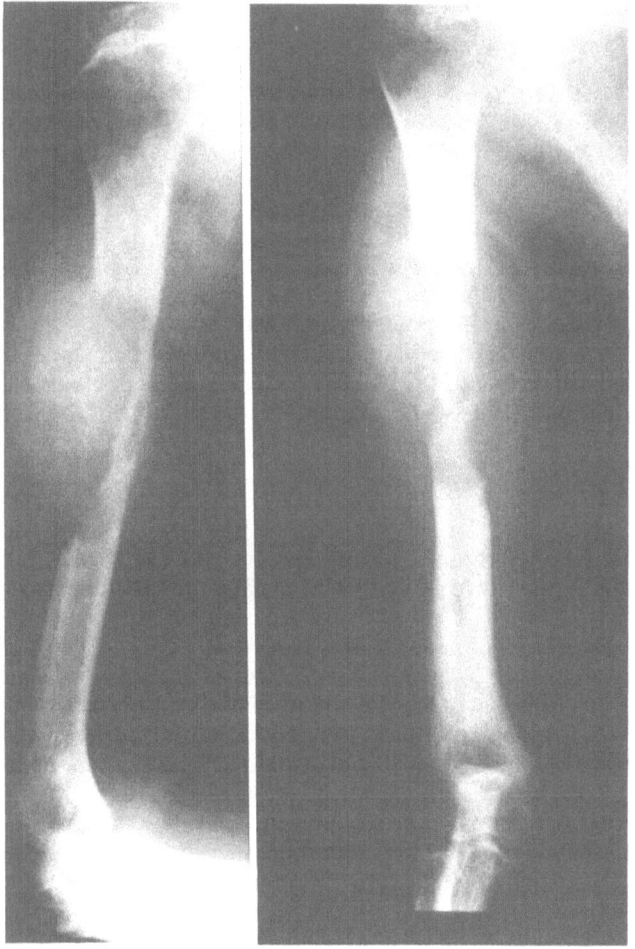

Fig. 11.4. Presenting lesion in a male patient with carcinoma of the kidney.

Post-operative irradiation of the renal bed (Finney 1974; Peeling et al. 1969) has been equally unrewarding and Bagshaw (1982b) believes that radiotherapy should be reserved for those in whom local excision is obviously incomplete in the hope that the incidence of local recurrences may be decreased.

Renal embolisation for inoperable tumours or in patients unfit for operation is a means of controlling troublesome haematuria and may have an immunological effect (MacErlean et al. 1980; Swanson et al. 1980). It may also be appropriate for the treatment of some lesions in patients with solitary kidneys. It is important to remember however that many renal tumours are relatively avascular and may be resistant to this approach; also that this technique is not without morbidity in terms of lumbar pain, malaise and fever over a period of 7–10 days, and that embolic complications have occurred from the presence of arterio-venous malformations within the tumour or from embolic material becoming displaced into the aorta and lodging elsewhere.

Hormone and Chemotherapy

Hormone therapy using medroxyprogesterone acetate (MPA) or testosterone (Bloom 1971) seemed promising but the early reports of 20% objective remissions have not been sustained and the literature since 1971 suggests that hormone treatment, whilst it may produce subjective relief, offers few objective responses (Hrushesky and Murphy 1977). Angioestrogens are also ineffective (Feun and Oishi 1979; Click et al. 1980). It seems illogical to continue to use such therapy since there is no evidence that renal tumours are hormone dependent. In addition it inhibits consideration of alternative forms of therapy.

Cytotoxic chemotherapy is equally disappointing, only vinblastine having shown activity (Hrushesky and Murphy 1977; Bodey 1979). Recent reports of the beneficial effect of the injection of tumour extracts (Tykkä et al. 1978; Neidhart et at. 1980a) offer hope for the future and merit further consideration.

EORTC Phase II Study

The EORTC Group has not so far felt it correct to establish any phase III studies, but has recently completed a phase II study of methyl-GAG in patients with measurable metastases of renal cancer (Child et al. 1982). This drug inhibits mitochondrial oxidation and suppresses polyamine synthesis (Mikles-Robertson et al. 1979; Porter et al. 1979). Methyl-GAG was given in a weekly dose of 500 mg/m² IV. Of 45 patients entered, 30 were evaluable for response, as they had received four or more treatment cycles. Of these, three (10%) achieved a partial remission by the World Health Organisation (WHO) criteria, i.e., more than 50% reduction in measurable tumour volume. The duration of response was from 8 to 12 weeks. Responses were observed in supraclavicular lymph nodes (two patients) and lung metastases (one patient). Toxicity was considerable and included nausea, vomiting, anorexia, muscle weakness, severe fatigue, arthralgia, and skin reactions. Six patients were taken off the study because of toxicity.

In view of the weak activity of methyl-GAG and the considerable toxicity encountered it cannot be recommended for use in renal cancer. The EORTC Group has now begun a study of vindesine in this disease.

Conclusions

Surgical excision of the primary lesion in the patient without metastases still offers the best hope of cure, a fact which emphasises the importance of early diagnosis and requires further education of the public and of the medical profession if this aim is to be achieved. Radiotherapy is probably best reserved for the palliation of residual or recurrent tumour in the renal fossa and for the treatment of non-resectable solitary metastases. Renal cancer is still peculiarly resistant to drugs and the role, if any, of immunotherapy awaits definition.

Testicular Tumours

Introduction

The management of seminoma of the testis by orchiectomy and subsequent radiotherapy to the regional lymph nodes yields a cure rate exceeding 90%. However, the 3-year survival of disseminated (stage III) seminoma averaged only 28% in the era before cisplatin-containing combination therapy (Caldwell et al. 1980). With the use of cisplatin, vinblastine and bleomycin (PVB) with or without adriamycin, Einhorn and Williams achieved 12/19 (63%) complete remissions. No patients had relapsed after a median follow-up of 18 months (Einhorn and Williams 1980a). Some European centres have had the same results (Cavalli et al. 1980). The major prognostic factor for the quality of response appeared to be the extent of metastatic disease. The results of chemotherapy in metastatic seminoma are similar to those achieved in non-seminomatous germ-cell tumours.

The therapeutic approach to the various stages of non-seminomatous tumours is much more complicated. In its consideration of testicular neoplasms, the EORTC Urological Group has confined its investigations to non-seminomatous lesions. The management of the different stages is summarised below. It is also recognised that the number of patients in any one centre or country is limited and it is hoped that cooperative studies will develop between the EORTC and the MRC in London.

Stage I Disease

The 5-year disease-free survival in clinical stage I disease exceeds 90% whether treatment after orchiectomy is by lymph node dissection or radiotherapy. It is conventional to treat the para-aortic nodes in all patients, as the failure rate for the detection of regional lymph node metastases using lymphography, CT scan, and markers is approximately 20%. Apparently, therefore, about 80% of the patients with clinical stage I have their radiotherapy or node dissection unnecessarily.

It is very tempting to suggest a 'wait and watch' policy after inguinal orchiectomy for patients with stage I disease. The main problem is the difficulty in evaluating the status of the retroperitoneal region at regular intervals. However, ultrasonography and CT scans are now practicable means for repeated screening.

In Britain the MRC is developing a study for clinical stage I testicular non-seminomas for patients with normal markers (β-HCG and alphafetoprotein) in serum and no evidence of tumour in the cut end of the spermatic cord in centres in London, Manchester, and Leeds and is hoping to collaborate in this and other studies with the EORTC. In Denmark a randomised study is being planned to compare radiotherapy (40 Gray in 4–5 weeks) versus no additional treatment after orchiectomy in stage I patients (DATECA Protocol 8004, HP Schultz 1981, personal communication), and in Norway and Sweden a study of unilateral versus bilateral node dissection in stage I patients was begun in March 1981 (SWENOTECA Protocol 1, SD Fossa 1981, personal communication).

Stage II Disease

Patients in this stage have lesions in the para-aortic nodes which may be easily resectable or in which the disease is so extensive as to make surgery difficult.

Einhorn (1979) reported on 52 patients with resectable stage II disease treated with orchiectomy and retroperitoneal node dissection. Eighteen of these patients (35%) developed metastases. All achieved complete remission with prompt combination chemotherapy. One patient relapsed and died and one died in complete remission of causes unrelated to cancer.

In patients with extensive stage II disease (patients with lymph node metastases larger than 2 cm) surgery frequently is difficult or impossible, and persistent disease is common following radiotherapy (Babaian and Johnson 1980). In addition, patients with extensive retroperitoneal disease run a high risk of developing haematogenous metastases (Edson 1980; Jacobs and Muggia 1980). Therefore the best treatment for extensive stage II disease is primary remission induction chemotherapy followed by retroperitoneal lymph node dissection in those patients who have evidence of residual tumour after induction treatment (Donohue et al. 1980; Babaian and Johnson 1980).

The case for and against radiotherapy, and for and against lymph node dissection, has been argued strongly, because the results of these modalities, whether used alone or in combination, have not proved entirely satisfactory. Although retroperitoneal dissection is accepted as the correct treatment for the para-aortic nodes in the United States and on the mainland of Europe, British oncologists still prefer to use radiotherapy as the treatment of choice. The question of the necessity for surgical intervention rather than radiotherapy as the first therapy remains unsolved, as it has never been subjected to randomised prospective clinical trial. However, the advantage of lymph node dissection is that it is a better staging procedure and more important that, unlike radiotherapy, it does not compromise later chemotherapy by provoking leukopenia and ileus when vinblastine is used.

Two years ago, the EORTC Urological Group considered and adopted four protocols designed to obtain further information in patients with stage II disease, recognising that the number of such patients was limited. The situation was further complicated by the commitment of some centres to lymph node dissection and of others to radiotherapy. The outline of the protocols was as follows:

1) For limited stage II disease
   (i) After radical bilateral retroperitoneal node dissection (Protocol 30791) or
   (ii) After radiologically diagnosed disease (Protocol 30793)
         — chemotherapy vs radiotherapy
2) For advanced stage II disease
   (i) After radical bilateral retroperitoneal node dissection (Protocol 30792) or
   (ii) After radiologically diagnosed disease (Protocol 30794)
         — chemotherapy vs radiotherapy + chemotherapy

The chemotherapeutic regime was the combination of *cis*-platinum, vinblastine, and bleomycin (PVB). Protocols 30791 and 30792 were never activated and unfortunately only three patients were entered to the remaining studies over a period of 18 months, as a result of which they have been closed to entry.

Advanced Disease

Combination Chemotherapy for Induction of Remission in Advanced Disease

Over the past few years, testicular non-seminomatous cancer has become a potentially curable disease. As a result of the development of highly active cisplatin-containing remission induction regimens, complete remissions are achieved in 60%–70% with a potential cure rate ranging from 45% to 60% (Cavalli et al. 1980; Bosl et al. 1980; Neidhart et al. 1980b; Newlands et al. 1980; Oliver et al. 1980; Samson et al. 1980; Scheulen et al. 1980a,b; Einhorn and Williams 1980b).

However, toxicity accompanying these regimens is considerable and 30%–55% of the patients do not achieve complete remission or relapse subsequently. Therefore, the research priorities are:

1) The reduction of the toxicity of these regimens without loss of activity;

2) Further increase in complete remission rates with new first line combination chemotherapy regimens;

3) The development of 'salvage' chemotherapy for patients failing first-line chemotherapy or relapsing subsequently; and

4) The evaluation of the necessity for, and duration of, maintenance chemotherapy.

The reduction of the dose of vinblastine from 0.4 to 0.3 mg/kg in the PVB regime by Einhorn and Williams (1980b) has led to a decrease from 35% to 15% of granulocytopenia and fever without decrease of activity.

In EORTC protocol 30795, patients with advanced testicular non-seminomas are randomised to receive PVB combination chemotherapy, comparing 0.4 mg to 0.3 of vinblastine, provided that these patients have not received previous radio- or chemotherapy. The end points of the study are complete remission rate, disease-free survival and overall survival. The incidence of agranulocytosis and fever in the two treatment groups will be related to these study parameters.

Patients who achieve a complete remission on this protocol are entered to the 'remission maintenance chemotherapy study' (EORTC Protocol 30796) which is described below.

Maintenance Chemotherapy in Advanced Disease

The value of maintenance chemotherapy is still undefined. Parallel to the situation in Hodgkin's disease, and gestational choriocarcinoma, several investigators feel that maintenance chemotherapy is unnecessary in patients with a well-documented complete remission because in such patients relapse hardly ever occurs. Patients who enter into complete remission only towards the end of the scheduled therapy may require longer induction treatment, e.g. six instead of four courses of PVB, to prevent relapse (Bosl et al. 1980). In the current EORTC trial (Protocol 30796) patients who attain a complete remission on Protocol 30795 (above) are randomised between cisplatin and vinblastine maintenance chemotherapy for 1 year compared to no maintenance therapy. Patients randomised to the chemotherapy arm receive vinblastine 0.2 mg/kg IV every 3 weeks and cisplatin 50 mg/m² IV every 6 weeks for 1 year.

Recent evidence (Einhorn et al. 1981) from a study in 113 patients suggests that maintenance therapy is unnecessary. There was a 9% relapse rate in 58 patients who received maintenance vinblastine, and a 7% relapse rate in 55 patients who were observed without treatment. Minimum follow-up was 1 year. These important results require confirmation.

Multimodality Treatment in Advanced Disease

Cytoreductive surgery may improve the results of chemotherapy in patients who present with bulky metastases. However, improvements in combination chemotherapy are so impressive that surgery has become adjunctive to chemotherapy.

The timing of debulking surgery remains a matter of debate. Large metastases at presentation may appear inoperable. Even if the volume can be reduced, new metastases may appear or rapid growth may occur during postoperative care. A 'sandwich' approach of initial chemotherapy of short duration followed by surgery and subsequent chemotherapy carries the risk of a long interval between chemotherapy cycles and therefore may have the same disadvantages.

Mathisen and Javadpour (1980) stressed that retroperitoneal tumour dissection is often extremely difficult and hazardous in patients with bulky abdominal metastases. In their recently completed NCI study of initial chemotherapy versus initial surgery followed by chemotherapy in patients with stage III testicular non-seminomas whose abdominal metastases were considered operable at the time of randomisation, they have developed a technique of en bloc resection of the inferior vena cava together with the tumour bulk to allow better access to the area behind the aorta. This enables more of the tumour to be removed and decreases the risk of major bleeding from injury to the vena cava or the aorta, and also lessens the risk of pulmonary embolism from clot or tumour located in the vena cava. However, analysis of the results showed that the procedure of initial surgery had a high morbidity, whereas these patients did not have a higher complete remission rate or a decreased relapse rate (Javadpour et al. 1981). This clearly shows that initial surgery does not benefit the patient.

When surgery is applied after the completion of induction chemotherapy, fibro-cystic elements are found in about one-third of the resected specimens, one-third will have mature teratomatous elements — still with malignant potential — and the remaining third will have persistent cancer including those with small malignant foci. Unless serum tumour markers are still elevated at the time of surgery, it is not possible to distinguish clinically between the three pathologic categories. Since it is important to recognise the patients with persistent cancer and mature teratoma for the planning of further treatment, all patients with clinical or roentgenographic evidence of residual masses at the completion of induction chemotherapy should be subjected to surgery.

Bearing in mind the disadvantages of initial or interim cytoreductive surgery as mentioned earlier, and looking at the excellent results of the study carried out by Donohue et al. (1980), supported by the observations of McLorie and Skinner (1980), the best approach to patients with far advanced disease seems to be initial remission induction chemotherapy followed by radical resection of residual tumour with additional induction chemotherapy for patients with persistent cancer in the resected specimen.

Salvage Chemotherapy

The development of re-induction chemotherapy or 'salvage' chemotherapy depends mainly on the identification of new active drugs. VP 16-213 (etoposide) has now been shown to be a very active drug in the treatment of testicular cancer, and at a dose of 100 mg/m^2 IV for 5 days, every 2–4 weeks, it gave an average remission rate of 40% in 76 patients with tumours refractory to chemotherapy (Dhafir et al. 1981; Fitzharris et al. 1980; Newlands and Bagshaw 1980). At Indiana University (Dhafir et al. 1981; Williams et al. 1980) 52 patients refractory to PVB, were treated with PVB + VP 16-213. A remission rate of 82% was achieved, 40% of which were complete remissions. The median survival of the responders was 52 weeks. Some of the complete responders are probably cured. Toxicity was considerable, with one drug-related death.

It appears that VP 16-213 is an essential component of 'salvage' chemotherapy regimens and its role in first-line combination chemotherapy is now being actively investigated in the United States and in Europe.

After the completion of its present testicular tumour studies, the EORTC Urological Group intends to implement further prospectively randomised studies to examine the value of remission induction regimens containing cisplatin–VP 16-213 in patients who have been pretreated and in those with a large tumour volume, since these are groups with a poor prognosis. In non-pretreated low tumour volume-bearing patients the group intends to study regimens with less toxicity than the PVB regimen.

Conclusions

The most important recent development in the treatment of advanced testicular cancer is the establishment of VP 16-213 as the second most active drug next to cisplatin. Future studies should include VP 16-213 in first-line regimens in an attempt to improve the cure rates.

There are increasing data to support the concept that maintenance chemotherapy is unnecessary for complete responders. Prolonged induction chemotherapy is, however, necessary for patients who enter complete remission late in the scheduled induction therapy.

In advanced disease cytoreductive surgery should be applied only to patients who, after remission induction treatment, have become marker-negative. Available data show that debulking surgery is useless in patients who still have active tumour.

Advanced stage II patients should be treated primarily with chemotherapy. Radiotherapy has no role to play, whereas lymph node dissection after chemotherapy is only necessary in patients who still have roentgenographic evidence of residual disease.

In stage I and stage II disease (nodes smaller than 2 cm) the standard approach is by retroperitoneal lymph node dissection or by radiotherapy. When dissection is performed and the nodes contain tumour cells, adjuvant chemotherapy may be given, but close observation of the patient for the development of metastases and subsequent chemotherapy is also justifiable. When the lymph nodes are negative a 'wait and watch' policy reserving chemotherapy for relapsing patients is also warranted.

Seminomas are as sensitive as teratomas to cisplatin-based chemotherapy and similar treatment strategies should be used in patients with advanced disease.

Acknowledgment. We are indebted to Mrs. S. Conyers without whose courtesy and cooperation this chapter would never have appeared.

References

Abbassian A, Wallace DM (1966) Intracavitary chemotherapy of diffuse non-infiltrating papillary carcinoma of the bladder. J Urol 96: 461–465

Altaffer LP III, Chenault ON Jr (1979) Paraneoplastic endocrinopathies associated with renal tumors. J Urol 122: 573–577

Auvert J, Botto H (1980) Treatment of malignant tumors of the bladder by iridium 192 wiring. In: Pavone-Macaluso M, Smith PH, Edsmyr F (eds) Bladder tumors and other topics in urological oncology. Plenum Press, London New York, pp 305–309

Babaian RJ, Johnson DE (1980) Management of stages I and II non-seminomatous germ tumors of the testis. Cancer 45: 1775–1781

Bagshaw MA (1982b) Radiotherapy of renal cancer: Principles and indications. In: Pavone-Macaluso M, Smith PH (eds) Cancer of the prostate and kidney. Plenum Press, London New York

Bagshaw MA (1982a) Radiotherapy of prostatic cancer. In: Pavone–Macaluso M, Smith PH (eds) Cancer of the prostate and kidney. Plenum Press, London New York

Beckley S, Wajsman Z, Slack N, Mittelman A, Murphy GP (1980) The chemotherapy of prostatic carcinoma. Scand J Urol Nephrol [Suppl] 55: 151–162

Bishop MC (1980) The treatment of bladder cancer with vitamin A. In: Pavone-Macaluso M, Smith PH, Edsmyr F (eds) Bladder tumors and other topics in urological oncology. Plenum Press, London New York pp 361–362

Blandy JP, England HR, Evans SJW, Hope-Stone HF, Mair GMM, Mantell BS, Oliver RTD, Paris AMI, Risdon RA (1980) T3 Bladder cancer — the case for salvage cystectomy. Br J Urol 152: 506–510

Bloom HJG (1971) Medroxyprogesterone acetate (Provera) in the treatment of metastatic renal cancer. Br J Cancer 25: 250–265

Bodey GP (1979) Current status of chemotherapy in metastatic renal carcinoma. In: Johnson DE, Samuels ML (eds) Cancer of the genito-urinary tract. Raven Press, New York, pp 67–72

Bosl GJ, Lange PH, Fraley EE (1980) Vinblastine, bleomycin and cis-diamminedichloroplatinum in the treatment of advanced testicular carcinoma. Possible importance of longer induction and shorter maintenance schedules. Am J Med 68: 492–496

Boxer RJ, Kaufman JJ, Goodwin WE (1977) Radical prostatectomy for carcinoma of the prostate: 1951–1976. A review of 329 patients. J Urol 117: 208–213

Burnand KG, Boyd PGR, Mayo ME, Shuttleworth KED, Lloyd-Davis RW (1976) Single-dose intra-vesical thio-tepa as adjuvant to cystodiathermy in the treatment of transitional cell bladder carcinoma. Br J Urol 48: 55–59

Byar D, Blackard C, VACURG (1977) Comparisons of placebo, pyridoxine and topical thiotepa in preventing recurrence of stage I bladder cancer. Urol 10: 556–561

Caldwell WL, Kademian T, Frias A, Davis E (1980) The management of testicular seminomas. Cancer 45: 1768–1774

Carmignani G, Belgrano E, Puppo P, Giberti C, Cichero A (to be published) Lymphadenectomy in renal cancer. In: Pavone–Macaluso M, Smith PH (eds) Cancer of the prostate and kidney. Plenum Press, London New York

Carter SK, Wasserman TH (1975) The chemotherapy of urologic cancer. Cancer 36: 729–747

Cavalli F, Monfardini S, Pizzocaro G (1980) Report of the international workshops on staging and treatment of testicular cancer. Eur J Cancer 16: 1367–1372

Child JA, Stoter G, Fossa SD, Bono AV, de Pauw M, EORTC Urological Group (to be published) Chemotherapy of advanced renal cell carcinoma. Results of treatment with methyl-glyoxal bis-guanylhydrazone (methyl-GAG); an EORTC study. In: Pavone-Macaluso M, Smith PH (eds) Cancer of the prostate and kidney. Plenum Press, London New York

Chisholm GD, Roy RR (1971) The systemic effects of malignant renal tumours. Br J Urol 43: 687–700

De Pauw M, Suciu S, Sylvester R, EORTC Genito-Urinary Tract Cooperative Group (1982) Preliminary results of two EORTC genito-urinary tract cooperative group protocols in previously untreated patients with T3–4 advanced prostatic cancer. In: Pavone–Macaluso M, Smith PH (eds) Cancer of the prostate and kidney. Plenum Press, London New York

Dhafir RA, Einhorn LH, Williams SD, Rosenbaum P, Issell B (1981) The effect of etoposide (VP-16), used alone or in combination on the survival of patients with refractory testicular cancer. Proc Am Soc Clin Oncol 22: 464

Donohue JP, Einhorn LH, Williams SD (1980) Cytoreductive surgery for metastatic testis cancer: considerations of timing and extent. J Urol 123: 876–880

Douville Y, Pelouze G, Roy R, Charrois R, Kibrité A, Martin M, Dionne L, Coulonval L, Robinson J (1978) Recurrent bladder papillomata treated with bacillus Calmette-Guérin: A preliminary report (Phase I trial). Cancer Treat Rep 62: 551–552

Edson M (1980) Testis cancer: the pendulun swings. Experience in 430 patients. J Urol 122: 763–765

Einhorn LH, Donohue J (1979) Adjuvant chemotherapy for testicular cancer: is it necessary? In: Jones SE, Salmon SE (eds) Proceedings of the Second International Conference on Adjuvant Therapy of Cancer, March 28–31, 1979, Tucson, Arizona, Grune & Stratton, New York pp 329–335

Einhorn LH, Williams SD (1980a) Chemotherapy of disseminated seminoma. Cancer Clin Trials 3: 307–313

Einhorn LE, Williams SD, (1980b) Chemotherapy of disseminated testicular cancer. A random prospective study. Cancer 46: 1339–1344

Einhorn LH, Williams SD, Troner M, Birch R, Grego FA (1981) The role of maintenance therapy in disseminated testicular cancer. New Engl J Med 305: 727–731

England HR, Molland EA, Oliver RTD, Blandy JP (1980a) Flat carcinoma in-situ of the bladder treated by systemic cyclophosphamide – a preliminary report. In: Pavone-Macaluso M, Smith PH, Edsmyr F (eds) Bladder tumors and other topics in urological oncology. Plenum Press, London New York, pp 371–376

England HR, Blandy JP, Paris AMI (1980b) The treatment of single and multiple papillary tumours of the bladder (Ta/T1 NX MO). In: Pavone-Macaluso M, Smith PH, Edsmyr F (eds) Bladder tumors and other topics in urological oncology. Plenum Press, London New York, pp 343–346

Feun LG, Oishi N (1979) Phase II study of nafoxidine in the therapy for advanced renal carcinoma. Cancer Treat Rep 63: 149–150

Finney R (1974) An evaluation of post-operative radiotherapy in hypernephroma treatment — a clinical trial. Cancer 32: 1332–1340

Fitzharris BM, Kaye SB, Saverymuttu S (1980) VP 16-213 as a single agent in advanced testicular tumors. Eur J Cancer 16: 1193–1197

Glick JH, Wein A, Torri S, Alavi J, Harris D, Brodovsky H (1980) Phase II study of tamoxifen in patients with advanced renal cell carcinoma. Cancer Treat Rep 64: 343–344

Hall RR (1980) Methotrexate therapy for multiple T1 Category bladder carcinoma. In: Pavone-Macaluso M, Smith PH, Edsmyr F (eds) Bladder tumors and other topics in urological oncology. Plenum Press, London New York, pp 377–380

Heaney JA, Chang HC, Daly JJ, Prout GR Jr (1977) Prognosis of clinically undiagnosed prostatic carcinoma and the influence of endocrine therapy. J Urol 118: 283–287

Helmstein K (1972) Treatment of bladder carcinoma by hydrostatic pressure technique: report of 43 cases. Br J Urol 44: 434–450

Houghton AL, Robinson MRG, Smith PH (1977) Melphalan in advanced prostatic cancer. A pilot study. Cancer Chemother Rep 61: 923–924

Hrushesky WJ, Murphy GP (1977) Current status of the therapy of advanced renal carcinoma. J Surg Oncol 9: 277–288

Jacobi GH, Kurth KH, Klippel KF, Hohenfellner R (1979) On the biological behaviour of T1-transitional cell tumours of the urinary bladder and initial results of the prophylactic use of topical adriamycin under controlled and randomised conditions. In: Diagnostics and treatment of superficial urinary bladder tumors. Montedison Läkemedel, Stockholn pp 83–94

Jacobs EM, Muggia FM (1980) Testicular cancer: risk factors and the role of adjuvant chemotherapy. Cancer 45: 1782–1790

Javadpour N, Ozols RF, Barlock A, Anderson T, Young RC (1981) A randomised trial of cytoreductive surgery followed by chemotherapy versus chemotherapy alone in bulky stage III testicular cancer. Proc Am Soc Clin Oncol 22–473

Kliman B, Prout GR Jr, Maclaughlin RA, Daly JJ, Griffin PP (1978) Altered androgen metabolism in metastatic prostate cancer. J Urol 119: 623–626

Lamm DL, Thor DE, Harris SC, Reyna JA, Stogdill VD, Radwin HM (1980) Bacillus Calmette-Guerin immunotherapy of superficial bladder cancer. J Urol 124: 38–42

Lund F (1969) Mucosal denudation (stripping) for bladder papillomatosis. Scand J Urol Nephrol 3: 204–207

McLorie GA, Skinner DG (1980) Metastatic non-seminomatous testis tumors: morbidity of treatment. J Urol 124: 479–481

McMillen SM, Wettlaufer JN (1976) The role of transurethral biopsy in Stage A carcinoma of the prostate. J Urol 116: 759–760

MacErlean DP, Owens AP, Bryan PJ (1980) Hypernephroma embolisation — is it worthwhile? Clin Radiol 31: 297–300

Martinez-Piñeiro JA (1980) BCG Vaccine in the treatment of non-infiltrating papillary tumours of the bladder. In: Pavone-Macaluso M, Smith PH, Edsmyr F (eds) Bladder tumours and other topics in urological oncology. Plenum Press, London New York: pp 175–185

Mathisen DJ, Javadpour N (1980) En bloc resection of inferior vena cava in cytoreductive surgery for bulky retroperitoneal metastatic testicular cancer. Urology 16: 51–54

Miklcs-Robertson F, Feurstein B, Dave C, Porter CW (1979) The generality of methylglyoxal bis(guanyl-hydrazone) induced mitochondrial damage and the dependence of this effect on cell proliferation. Cancer Res 39: 1919–1926

Morales A, Eidinger D, Bruce AW (1976) Intracavitary bacillus Calmette-Guérin in the treatment of superficial bladder tumors. J Urol 116: 180–183

Neidhart JA, Murphy SG, Hennick LA, Wise HA (1980a) Active specific immunotherapy os stage IV renal carcinoma with aggregated tumor antigen adjuvant. Cancer 46: 1128–1134

Neidhart JA, Memo R, Metz EN (1980b) Probable cure of metastatic testicular tumors treated with sequential therapy. Cancer Treat Rep 64: 553–558

Newlands ES, Bagshaw KD (1980) Antitumour activity of the epipodophyllin derivative VP 16-213 (etoposide: NSC-141540) in gestational choriocarcinoma. Eur J Cancxer 16: 401–405

Newlands ES, Begent RHJ, Kaye SB (1980) Chemotherapy of advanced malignant teratomas. Br J Cancer 42: 378–384

Oliver RTD, Ama Rohatinet A, Wrigley PFM, Malpas JS (1980) Chemotherapy of metastatic testicular tumours. Br J Urol 52: 34–37

Pavone-Macaluso M (1979) Intravesical treatment of superficial (T1) urinary bladder tumours — a review of a 15-year experience. In: Diagnostics and treatment of superficial urinary bladder tumors. Montedison Läkemedel, Stockholm, pp 21–36

Peeling WB, Mantell BS, Shepheard BGF (1969) Post-operative irradiation in the treatment of renal cell carcinoma. Br J Urol 41: 23–31

Porter CW, Mikles-Robertson D, Kramer D, Dave C (1979) Correlation of ultrastructural and functional damage to mitochondria of ascites L1210 cells treated in vivo with methylglyoxal bis(guanylhydrazone) or ethidium bromide. Cancer Res 39: 2414–2421

Prout GR Jr (1977) The role of surgery in the potentially curative treatment of bladder carcinoma. Cancer Res 37: 2764–2770

Prout GR Jr (1981) The philosophy of national bladder cancer project studies. In: Denis L, Smith PH, Pavone-Macaluso M (eds) Clinical bladder cancer. Plenum Press, London New York

Samson MK, Fisher R, Stephens RL (1980) Vinblastine, bleomycin and cis-diamminedichloroplatinum in disseminated testicular cancer: response to treatment and prognostic correlations. Eur J Cancer 1359–1366

Scheulen ME, Higi M, Schilcher RB (1980a) Sequentiell alternierende Chemotherapie nicht Semino-matöser Hodentumoren mit Velbe, Bleomycin und Adriamycin/Cisplatin. Klin Wochenschr 58: 811–821

Scheulen ME, Seeber S, Schilcher RB (1980b) Sequential combination chemotherapy with vinblastine, bleomycin and doxorubicin, cis-dichlorodiammine platinum (II) in disseminated non-seminomatous testicular cancer. Cancer Treat Rep 64: 599–609

Schmidt JD (to be published) Chemotherapy of prostate cancer: The National Prostatic Cancer Project (NPCP) experience. In: Pavone-Macaluso M, Smith PH (eds) Cancer of the prostate and kidney. Plenum Press, London New York

Schroeder FH, Belt E (1975) Carcinoma of the prostate: a study of 213 patients with stage C tumors treated by total perineal prostatectomy. J Urol 114: 257–260

Schulman CC, EORTC Urological Group (1980) Adjuvant therapy of T1 bladder carcinoma: preliminary results of an EORTC randomised study. In: Pavone-Macaluso M, Smith PH, Edsmyr F (eds) Bladder tumors and other topics in urological oncology. Plenum Press, London New York, pp 347–354

Schlegel JU, Pipkin GE, Nishimura R, Schultz GN (1970) The role of ascorbic acid in the prevention of bladder tumour formation. J Urol 103: 155–159

Smith PH (180) The medical management of prostatic cancer — some current questions. Eur Urol 6: 65–68

Smith PH (1981a) Adjuvant chemotherapy in bladder cancer. J R Soc Med 74: 547–550

Smith PH (1981b) Endocrine and cytotoxic therapy. In: Duncan W (ed) Prostate Cancer, Springer-Verlag, Berlin, Heidelberg and New York, pp 154–172

Sternberg JJ, Bracken RB, Handel PB, Johnson DE (1977) Combination therapy (CISCA) for advanced urinary tract carcinoma. JAMA 238: 2282–2287

Swanson DA, Wallace S, Johnson DE (1980) The role of embolization and nephrectomy in the treatment of metastatic renal carcinoma. Urol Clin North A 7: 719–729

Tykkä H, Oravisto KJ, Lehtonen T, Sarna S, Tallberg T (1978) Active specific immunotherapy of advanced renal cell carcinoma. Eur Urol 4: 250–258

Veterans Administration Cooperative Urological Research Group (1967) Treatment and survival of patients with cancer of the prostate. Surg Gynecol Obstet 124: 1011–1017

Wallace DM, Bloom HJG (1976) The management of deeply infiltrating (T3) bladder carcinoma: con-trolled trial of radical radiotherapy versus pre-operative radiotherapy and radical cystectomy (first report). Br J Urol 48: 587–594

Weaver PC, Learmonth ID, Lloyd Thomas T, Hutter BF, Cox R, Dixon Sir P (1979) Advanced bladder carcinoma treated by cystectomy: a report on twenty-three years experience (with special reference to salvage cystectomy following radical radiotherapy). Clin Oncol 5: 3–9

Werf-Messing B van der (1980) Carcinoma of the urinary bladder treated by interstitial radium implant. In: Pavone-Macaluso M, Smith PH, Edsmyr F (eds) Bladder tumors and other topics in urological oncology. Plenum Press, London New York, pp 311–312

Werf-Messing B van der, Heul R O van der Ledeboer RC (1978) Renal cell carcinoma trial. Cancer Clin Trials 13–21

Williams SD, Einhorn LH, Greco FA (1980) VP16-213 salvage therapy for refractory germinal neoplasm. Cancer 46: 2154–2158

Appendix: EORTC Studies in Progress

Protocols Closed to Entry

a) Bladder Cancer

30751 — Phase III trial comparing intravesical thiotepa (30 mg) vs VM26 (50 mg) vs no additional treatment after complete transurethral resection (TUR) of all lesions in patients with category T1 bladder cancer. Closed to entry October 1978 with 294 evaluable patients.

30764 — Phase II study of cyclophosphamide (1000 mg/m^2) *or* adriamycin (75 mg/m^2 *or* adriamycin (50 mg/m^2) plus 5-fluorouracil (500 mg/m^2) in patients with advanced bladder cancer. Closed entry because of poor recruitment November 1978 with 34 evaluable patients.

30771 — Advanced bladder cancer. Phase II trial of *cis*-platinum (cisplatin) (40 mg/m^2), adriamycin (40 mg/m^2) and cyclophosphamide (400 mg/m^2) given in 3-weekly cycles. Closed to entry June 1980 with 44 evaluable patients.

30784 — Category T3 bladder cancer. Phase III trial comparing treatment with adriamycin (40 mg/m^2) + 5-fluorouracil (500 mg/m^2) vs no additional treatment after radical cystectomy with or without pre-operative flash radiotherapy. Closed to entry March 1981 because of inadequate recruitment.

b) Prostatic Cancer

30761 — Phase III trial comparing cyproterone acetate (250 mg daily), medroxy-progesterone acetate (500 mg IM three times a week for 8 weeks, then 100 mg orally b.d.) and stilboestrol (1 mg t.d.s.) in T3 T4, MO, and TO-4, M1 prostatic cancer. Closed to entry March 1981 with 296 currently evaluable patients.

30762 — Phase III trial comparing estracyt (280 mg b.d. for 8 weeks + 140 mg b.d. thereafter) and stilboestrol (1 mg t.d.s.) in the same categories of patients as 30761. Closed to entry June 1980 with 248 evaluable patients.

30763 — Phase II study of adriamycin (60 mg/m^2 every 3 weeks) and of pro-carbazine (200 mg/m^2 days 1–14 of each 28-day cycle). Closed to entry June 1979 because of toxicity encountered with procarbazine.

c) Renal Cancer

30801 — Phase II study of methyl-GAG (500 mg/m^2 IV weekly) in metastatic renal cancer. Closed March 1981 with 40 evaluable patients.

Active Protocols (patients entered up to July 1981)

a) Bladder Cancer

30781 — Phase III trial of pyridoxine (20 mg daily) vs placebo in patients with category Ta/T1 bladder cancer to assess incidence of recurrence after complete TUR of all visible lesions. Since January 1979 253 patients entered.

30782 — Phase III trial of intravesical adriamycin (50 mg) vs cisplatin (50 mg) vs thiotepa (50 mg) in patients with recurrent category Ta/T1 bladder cancer after complete TUR. Since March 1979 207 patients have been entered.

30790 — Phase III trial of intravesical epodyl (1.13 g) vs adriamycin (50 mg) vs no additional treatment following complete TUR of category Ta/T1 lesions either new or recurrent. Since December 1979 141 patients have been entered.

30797 — Phase II study of vincristine (1 mg/m^2 weekly) in patients with advanced bladder cancer with measurable metastases. Forty-three patients entered since February 1979 (entry restricted to those not eligible for entry to protocols 30771 or 30802).

30802 — Phase II study of cisplatin (70 mg/m^2 on day 1) + VM26 (100 mg/m^2 day 1 + 2) every 3 weeks in patients with bladder cancer with measurable metastases. Twenty-eight patients entered since 1980.

b) Prostatic Cancer

30805 — Phase III trial of stilboestrol (1 mg daily) vs orchiectomy vs orchiectomy and cyproterone acetate (50 mg t.d.s.). Activated June 1981.

30799 — Phase II study of vindesine (3 mg/m^2 weekly) in patients with measurable metastatic disease resistant to conventional treatment. Thirty-nine patients entered since August 1979.

c) Testicular Cancer

30795 — Induction of remission with cisplatin, bleomycin and vinblastine in patients with advanced non-seminoma. Patients receive CDDP 20 mg/m^2 IV days 1–5 every 3 weeks and bleomycin 30 mg IV day 2 then weekly times 12. In addition, they are randomised either to receive vinblastine 0.20 mg/kg IV day 1–2 every 3 weeks (100% VBL) or vinblastine 0.15 mg/kg IV day 1–2 every 3 weeks (75% VBL). Since February 1979 131 patients have been entered.

30796 — Following complete remission induction patients are randomised between maintenance therapy with vinblastine (0.2 mg/kg IV every 3 weeks) + cisplatin (50 mg/m^2 IV every 6 weeks) and no additional treatment. Thirty-eight patients have entered this study since obtaining complete remission in 30795.

Chapter 12

Future Progress in Chemotherapy of Urological Tumors

A. S. D. Spiers

In the preceding chapters, several of the authors have indicated likely future developments in their respective fields. While the increasing effort in basic and clinical research seems to assure that there will be advances in the chemotherapeutic management of the urological tumors, it is difficult to predict either the rate or the extent of progress. Experience suggests that it will be neither very rapid nor very dramatic: 'breakthroughs' are common in the media but rare in the real world of clinical science.

Caution is also necessary in attempting to predict the avenues of research that will lead to progress. Scientifically, the most appealing approach is that of learning more about the biology of urological tumors, including the intimate details of their cellular chemistry and cell:cell interactions, so that a 'rational' therapy can be devised for each tumor. Further refinement might disclose criteria by which appropriate therapy can be selected for each patient. It must be acknowledged that this approach in cancer research, while contributing much to our understanding of cellular and sub-cellular processes, has contributed little to practical bedside therapeutics. On occasion, it has explained why certain empirically derived treatments do in fact work, but it has not been notably successful in suggesting new lines of treatment which then are shown to be effective. Therapeutic experimentation, despite an often tenuous rationale, usually has been more productive.

The empirical approach, assessing a whole series of agents in each tumor, is cumbersome, time consuming, and expensive. In some instances — for example renal carcinoma — it has been relatively unrewarding. True, there is always the possibility of a new agent with a high degree of activity 'turning up', but this Micawberish expectation seems less likely to be fulfilled than it did in the 1950s, when chemotherapy was in its infancy. With a few exceptions, notably cisplatin, most of the advances of the last decade have been made by the improved use of existing agents, rather than the discovery of new drugs. Several of the authors have pointed out that for most urological cancers there is a paucity of reliable data concerning the effectiveness even of standard agents that have been available for many years. This deficit is being remedied by the cooperative group studies now in progress, and by the planning of new studies which will examine old and new drugs, and will test chemotherapy both for metastatic disease and as an adjunct to surgery or radio-therapy. Even when the gains from chemotherapy are modest, cooperative group studies offer tangible advantages: (a) the existence of a formal trial tends to standardize, and to improve, the quality of care; (b) well-designed trials frequently contribute valuable additional knowledge on the natural history of the tumors concerned; (c) a mechanism is created whereby new ideas — often the result of single-institution pilot studies — can be evaluated in a relatively short period, so that genuine advances are verified rapidly and then made available for more widespread use.

In adrenal cancer, improved methods for detecting early disease are needed. The unique properties of mitotane (o,p'-DDD) suggest the desirability of testing further structural analogues of this compound. As in all the rarer urological cancers, cooperative studies should have high priority, to enable the completion of drug trials in a reasonable period of time. A recent report (Tattersall et al. 1980) describes clinical and objective responses in all of four patients with metastatic adrenal cancer who received cisplatin. One of my patients with rapidly progressive adrenal cancer has had stabilization of disease for 7 months with the same treatment. Clearly, cisplatin merits more extensive evaluation in adrenal cancer.

Carcinoma of the kidney has proved remarkably resistant to cytotoxic drugs of any type. The principal contribution of many clinical trials has been to demonstrate the ineffectiveness of both cytotoxic agents and hormones. This has undoubted value, as patients will in future be spared toxic and futile therapy, and a further stimulus is provided for therapeutic research. Because of the capricious nature of renal cancer, studies with cancer chemotherapeutic agents require groups of patients who receive no specific therapy: there is in this tumor no ethical objection to this experimental design, as there is no standard therapy of proved value. Methyl-glyoxal-bisguanyl-hydrazone appears to possess modest activity in renal cancer, and experience with this drug needs to be enlarged; it is at present unjustified to incorporate it into a multiple-drug regimen, but a surgical adjuvant study should be mounted. Available nephro-toxic agents may be screened in vitro, or against tumor implants in nude mice, for activity against renal cancer, and promising agents might be administered to patients with metastatic renal cancer while their healthy kidney is maintained on an extra-corporeal circuit. Unfortunately, the nephrotoxicity of many drugs and chemicals may well depend on the normal physiological activity of renal tissue, and patho-logical renal tissue may not be similarly susceptible. Thus cisplatin, which is a potent nephrotoxin unless special precautions are taken, seems ineffective in carcinoma of the kidney.

In contrast, Kumar and his colleagues are able to report impressive advances in the management of Wilms' tumor. Further progress is to be expected from more precise clinical and pathological staging, from improved techniques of radionuclide imaging, and from more refined surgical techniques. Wilms' tumor is responsive to a wide range of drugs, but the emergence of drug-resistant tumor cells accounts for a significant number of therapeutic failures. The systematic screening of new agents for activity in Wilms' tumor should have high priority.

Progress in the management of the rarer tumors of the urothelium — the renal pelvis, ureter, and urethra — is likely to be brought about by collaborative studies. No single institution can accrue, in any reasonable time span, sufficient patients to conduct even a simple two-armed study. Fundamental questions, for example the efficacy (or otherwise) of preoperative or postoperative radiotherapy, are un-answered. Adjuvant chemotherapy cannot reasonably be studied, because chemo-therapeutic agents with sufficient activity have not yet been identified.

In bladder cancer, several agents are known to possess useful activity: this opens the way for surgical adjuvant studies. For metastatic bladder cancer, trials of single-agent versus multiple-agent chemotherapy are in progress, and there is a need to continue the screening of new agents. The observation (Falor and Ward 1976; 1978) that cytogenetic studies of urothelial cells may be of value in the prognosis of early bladder cancer, indicating those patients who are at high risk of recurrence and invasive disease, and in whom early radical excision should be considered, merits further evaluation. As the treatment of advanced bladder cancer must still be considered very unsatisfactory, the detection of high-risk patients among those with early tumors is of special importance.

Several cooperative trials are assessing the role of drug therapy in carcinoma of the prostate. The advent of useful cytotoxic therapy for this tumor will diminish the role of hormone therapy, with its undoubted side effects and limited benefits. The development of hormone receptor assays that are applicable to prostatic tissue offers the possibility that in future, orchiectomy or the administration of androgen antagonists or estrogens may be selected rationally, rather than tried empirically, with a resultant higher success rate, as is now achieved in breast cancer. An empirical trial of tamoxifen in prostatic cancer, carried out by the Eastern Cooperative Oncology Group appears, on preliminary analysis, to have negative results. The advent of a hormone receptor assay which reliably predicts those patients who will not benefit from hormonal manipulations, would avoid needless trials of ineffective therapy, and these patients would have the opportunity for an earlier trial of cytoxic drugs only after a trial of hormone therapy, and frequently after radiotherapy also, and are in poor general condition. This prejudices their chances of response, and may also invalidate the assessment of the chemotherapeutic regimen under study.

Recent findings of interest in cancer of the prostate include the demonstration that aminoglutethimide, and antagonist of steroid synthesis by the adrenals, is active in patients with metastatic disease, and may be effective when disease progression has occurred after orchiectomy (Robinson 1980; Worgul et al. 1981). A preliminary report suggests that a combination of doxorubicin, mitomycin C and 5-fluorouracil is highly active in advanced prostatic cancer (Logothetis et al. 1981). We have found this combination to be active, but dose reductions are necessary, particularly in patients who have received previous radiotherapy.

In testicular cancer, as in Wilms' tumor, advances will be made in two divergent ways. Current studies of pathology, stage, and outcome will enable the future identification of 'good risk' patients who will be cured by less aggressive therapy, with lesser morbidity from treatment. This will be a significant advance, as curative therapy for testicular cancer can produce severe physical and psychological impairment, as one articulate patient has so well pointed out (Fiore 1979). At the other end of the scale, better therapy is needed for the 'poor risk' patients who develop metastatic disease, and later, refractoriness to the best chemotherapeutic agents. Trial of new agents is the standard approach to this problem, but much greater refinement will be attained if recently developed techniques of clonogenic assay for the sensitivity of tumor cells in vitro to cytotoxic drugs (Salmon et al. 1978) can be applied to material from germ-cell tumors of the testis.

Advances in vascular radiology will contribute to the chemotherapy of urological cancers. It is technically possible to catheterize percutaneously the arterial supply of primary tumors and also that of major metastases, and to deliver cytotoxic drugs directly into the vascular bed of tumor masses. This approach is not new, but has suffered from a lack of controlled clinical trials, with resulting justifiable scepticism regarding its value. In the modern era of chemotherapy, with more informed choices of drug, dose, and schedule, intra-arterial chemotherapy merits re-evaluation. Recent results in the local control of breast cancer (Stephens et al. 1980) might well be equalled, or surpassed, in renal or adrenal cancer.

The key to future progress in the management of urological cancers will be cooperation. This implies not only the multi-institutional cooperative group, which makes possible the rapid accrual of cases and the speedy evaluation of new therapies. There will also be progress because of interdisciplinary collaboration within institutions, patients being assessed by a team which includes the urologist, medical oncologist, radiotherapist, radiologist, and pharmacologist, so that multimodality therapy can be planned from the outset. The team approach, combined with the critical appraisal of results and the willingness to adopt new strategies, will bring about significant benefits for the patient with urological cancer.

References

Falor WH, Ward RM (1976) Cytogenetic analysis: a potential index for recurrence of early carcinoma of the bladder. J Urol 115: 49–52

Falor WH, Ward RM (1978) Prognosis in early carcinoma of the bladder based on chromosomal analysis. J Urol 119: 44–47

Fiore N (1979) Fighting cancer—one patient's perspective. N Engl J Med 300: 284–289

Logothetis C, von Eschenbach A, Samuels M, Haynie TP, Johnson DE (1981) Doxorubicin, mitomycin-C, 5-fluorouracil (DMF) in the therapy of hormonal resistant adenocarcinoma of the prostate. Proc Am Soc Clin Oncol 22: 462, C-507

Robinson M (1980) Aminoglutethimide: medical adrenalectomy in the management of carcinoma of the prostate. Br J Urol 52: 328–329

Salmon SE, Hamburger AW, Soehnlen B, Durie GM, Alberts DS, Moon TE (1978) Quantitation of differential sensitivity of human tumor stem cells to anticancer drugs. N Engl J Med 298: 1321–1327

Stephens FO, Crea P, Harker GJS, Roberts BA, Hambly CK (1980) Intra-arterial chemotherapy as basal treatment in advanced and fungating primary breast cancer. Lancet II: 435–438

Tatterstall MHN, Lander H, Bain B et al. (1980) Cis-platinum treatment of metastatic adrenal carcinoma. Med J Aust 1: 419–421

Worgul TJ, Santen RJ, Samojlik E, Lipton A, Harvey H, Veldhuis JD, Drago JR, Rohner TJ (1981) Clinical and biochemical effect of aminoglutethimide in the treatment of advanced prostatic carcinoma. Proc Am Soc Clin Oncol 22: 471, C-542

Appendix

Major cytotoxic agents referred to in the text [1,2,3]

Generic name	Proprietary[4] and other names	Usual[5] route	Mode of action	Major[6,7,8] toxicity	Precautions[9] for handling	Comments
Bleomycin	Blenoxane	IV	Cleavage of DNA	CU	Wear gloves, avoid inhalation	Not toxic to bone marrow. Severe pulmonary fibrosis
Carmustine	BiCNU; BCNU	IV	Alkylating agent	BM, NV, TP	Avoid skin contact	Causes protracted marrow depression, thrombocytopenia
Chlorambucil	Leukeran	PO	Alkylating agent	BM	None	Long-term administration erodes marrow function
Cisplatin	Platinol; DDP; cis-DDP; cis-platinum II	IV	Probably an alkylating agent	NV	Avoid skin contact	Ototoxic; nephrotoxic; may potentiate other nephrotoxic agents
Cyclophosphamide	Cytoxan; Endoxana; CTX; CPM	IV PO	Alkylating agent	BM, NV, AL	None	Severe haemorrhagic cystitis
Dacarbazine	DTIC; dimethyl-triazeno-imidazole carboxamide	IV	Probably an alkylating agent	BM, NV, AL, PN	Wear gloves	Occasional flulike syndrome: fever, myalgia, beginning about day 7; lasts 1–3 weeks
Dactinomycin	Cosmegen; DACT; actinomycin D	IV	Binds to DNA helix	BM, NV, AL, CE, MU, CU	Wear gloves	Recurrent erythema in old radiotherapy fields
Doxorubicin	Adriamycin; hydroxy-daunorubicin	IV	Binds to DNA helix	BM, NV, AL, CE, TP, MU	Wear gloves	Severe cardiotoxicity. Dose reduction in liver disease
Estramustine	Estracyt	PO IV	Alkylating; estrogenic	NV, TP	None	Fluid retention, heart failure, gynecomastia
Ethoglucid	Epodyl	IV IC	Alkylating agent	NV, BM	Wear gloves	Hypotension and faintness for 2 minutes after injection

Appendix Major cytotoxic agents referred to in the text

Generic name	Proprietary[4] and other names	Usual[5] route	Mode of action	Major[6,7,8] toxicity	Precautions[9] for handling	Comments
Etopside	VP16-213; epipodophyllotoxin	IV	Inhibits mitosis and DNA synthesis	BM, AL	Avoid skin contact	Headache, fever, hypotension, bronchospasm
5-Fluorouracil	Adrucil; 5-FU	IV	Pyrimidine antimetabolite	BM, MU D, CN	None	Occasional vomiting, headache cerebellar ataxia
Lomustine	CeeNU; CCNU	PO	Alkylating agent	BM, NV	None	Nephrotoxic with prolonged use. Rare confusion, ataxia
Melphalan	Alkeran; phenyl-alanine mustard	PO	Alkylating agent	BM, NV	None	Probably leukaemogenic. Rare pulmonary fibrosis
Methotrexate	Mexate; amethopterin	PO IV	Folic acid antagonist	BM, AL, MU, D	Avoid skin contact	Hepatocellular injury, obstructive nephropathy with high dose regimens
Methyl-GAG	MGBG; methyl-glyoxal-bis-guanylhydrazone	IV	Antagonizes polyamine synthesis	MU, CU, D	None	Pharyngitis, esophagitis, proctitis, hypoglycemia, vasculitis, anemia
Mithramycin	Mithracin; aureolic acid	IV	Binds to DNA helix	BM, NV, D MU, CU, CN	None	Hemorrhage due to lowering platelet count and Factors II, V, VII, and X: may be fatal
Mitomycin	Mutamycin; mitomycin C	IV	Alkylating agent	BM, TP, CE	Wear gloves	Purple bands in nail beds. drowsiness, fever, rare renal and pulmonary toxicity
Mitotane	Lysodren; o'p'-DDD	PO	Uncertain	NV, D, CN	None	Lethargy, depression, vertigo, adrenal insufficiency
Nitrogen mustard	Mustargen; HN2; mechlorethamine HCl	IV	Alkylating agent	BM, NV, TP, CE	Wear gloves	Rare allergic reactions, mucositis
Thiotepa	Thio-Tepa; triethylene thiophosphoramide	IV IC	Alkylating agent	BM	Avoid skin contact	Nausea, vomiting, dizziness, headache, allergy — all rare

Appendix Major cytotoxic agents referred to in the text

Generic name	Proprietary[4] and other names	Usual[5] route	Mode of action	Major[6,7,8] toxicity	Precautions[9] for handling	Comments
Vinblastine	Velban; Velbe; vincaleukoblastine	IV	Mitotic inhibition	BM, C, PN, AL, TP, CE	Wear gloves	Nausea, vomiting, rashes, mucositis — all uncommon
Vincristine	Oncovin; VCR	IV	Mitotic inhibition	PN, CN, AL, C, TP, CE	Wear gloves	Severe peripheral neuropathy, inappropriate ADH secretion, hypotension, paralytic ileus

[1] This list is not comprehensive. Agents mentioned only once or twice in the text are omitted.

[2] Doses are not included because these vary with the schedule of administration, the inclusion of other cytotoxic agents in the treatment regimen, and with factors in individual patients — for example, previous treatment, liver disease.

[3] All these compounds have significant toxicity and should be administered by physicians experienced in their use.

[4] Proprietary names appear first. Not all these compounds are commercially available.

[5] IV = intravenous; PO = by mouth; IC = intracavitary or intraluminal.

[6] Key: CU = cutaneous; BM = marrow depression; NV = nausea, vomiting; TP = thrombophlebitis; AL = alopecia; PN = peripheral nervous system; CE = cellulitis with extravasation; MU = mucositis; D = diarrhea; CN = central nervous system; C = constipation. Toxic effects are listed for each drug in their approximate order of importance.

[7] A toxic effect is not listed if it is uncommon with the agent concerned. This does not mean it is never observed.

[8] Toxic effects special to individual drugs, or of special importance, are listed under *Comments*.

[9] In general, these are those recommended by the manufacturers.

References

Dorr RT, Fritz WL (1980) Cancer chemotherapy handbook. Elsevier, New York Oxford

Knowles RS, Virden JE (1980) Handling of injectable antineoplastic agents. Br Med J 280: 589—591

Subject Index

from the series
Recent Results in Cancer Research

Cancer Chemo- and Immunopharmacology
In two parts

Volume 74: Part 1:
Chemopharmacology
Editors: G. Mathé, F. M. Muggia

1980. 82 figures, 150 tables. XIII, 315 pages
ISBN 3-540-10162-4

Volume 75: Part 2:
Immunopharmacology, Relations, and General Problems
Editors: G. Mathé, F. M. Muggia

1980. 76 figures, 83 tables. XI, 260 pages
ISBN 3-540-10163-2

Volume 76
New Drugs in Cancer Chemotherapy
Editors: S. K. Carter, Y. Sakurai, H. Umezawa

1981. 133 figures, 170 tables. XIV, 336 pages
ISBN 3-540-10487-9

Volume 78:
Prostate Cancer
Editor: W. Duncan

1981. 68 figures, 67 tables. X, 190 pages
ISBN 3-540-10676-6

Volume 80:
Adjuvant Therapies of Cancer
Editors: G. Mathé, G. Bonadonna, S. E. Salmon

1982. 108 figures, 146 tables. XVI, 356 pages
ISBN 3-540-10949-8

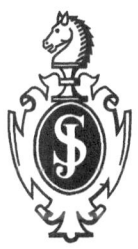

Springer-Verlag
Berlin
Heidelberg
New York

Renal and Adrenal Tumors

Pathology, Radiology, Ultrasonography, Therapy, Immunology

Editor: E. Löhr
In collaboration with numerous experts
Translated in Part from the German by H.-U. Eickenberg
1979. 209 figures (14 in color) in 344 separate illustrations,
42 tables. XVIII, 372 pages.
ISBN 3-540-09192-0

Idiopathic Hydronephrosis

Editors: P. H. O'Reilly, J. A. Gosling
Foreword by E. C. Edwards
1982. 87 figures. XII, 132 pages
ISBN 3-540-10937-4

W. W. Park

The Histology of Borderline Cancer

With Notes on Prognosis

With the collaboration of J. W. Corkhill
1980. 314 figures, 21 tables. XIV, 471 pages
ISBN 3-540-09792-9

The Ureter

Editor: H. Bergmann
With 52 Contributors
2nd edition. 1981. 760 figures. XVII, 780 pages
ISBN 3-540-90561-8

A. T. K. Cockett, K. Koshiba

Manual of Urologic Surgery

Illustrated by J. Takamoto

1979. 532 color illustrations. XVIII, 284 pages
(Comprehensive Manuals of Surgical Specialties)
ISBN 3-540-90423-9

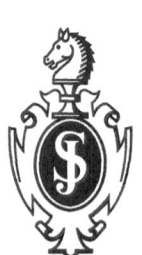

Springer-Verlag
Berlin
Heidelberg
New York

Surgery of Female Incontinence

Editors: S. L. Stanton, E. A. Tanagho
With a Foreword by Sir John Dewhurst
1980. 199 figures, 17 tables. XVI, 203 pages
ISBN 3-540-10155-1